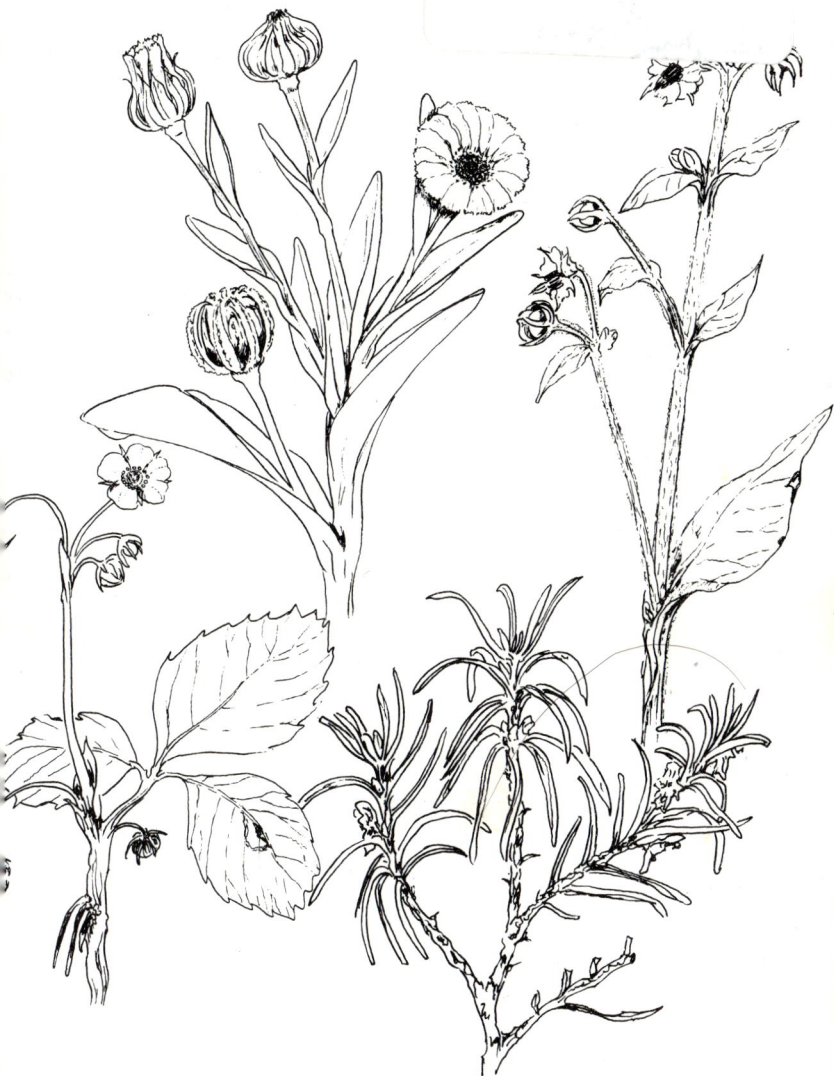

Health
from the
Hedgerow

Health from the Hedgerow

A naturalist's encyclopaedia of medicinal plants

Dennis Furnell

B. T. BATSFORD LTD
LONDON

For Ann

ISBN 0 7134 4712 5 (cased)

Typeset by Keyspools Ltd, Golborne, Lancs
and printed in Great Britain by
Butler & Tanner Ltd
Frome, Somerset
for the publishers
B. T. Batsford Ltd
4 Fitzhardinge Street
London W1H 0AH

Contents

Acknowledgements

I would like to thank several people for the assistance and support they gave me during the research and production of this book.

Trevor Wade, who encouraged me to begin by commissioning the original articles for the *Evening Post and Echo*, for his enthusiasm that I should turn the results of my research into a book.

Reg Smith of the Hawk Conservancy, whose assistance in finding additional reference sources was invaluable.

The editor and staff of *Here's Health* for their support.

Jack Harpley for his friendly assistance in giving me plant seeds and for his knowledge generously offered.

The directors and staff of Bushey Colour Laboratories Co., Ltd for technical assistance in the processing of colour photographs for this book and for providing friendly personal service, even though I was very demanding.

Gordon Mellor, FPS, for pointing me in the direction of the *Pharmaceutical Handbook* and for objective support and advice.

The Hon. David Lytton Cobbold for permission to use the photograph of Gertrude Jekyll's herb garden at Knebworth House (back of jacket).

Cyril Lane for his help in finding some of the wild plants I wanted to photograph.

Sharon Venes, whose cheerful attitude to the seemingly endless task of drafting and re-drafting the manuscript was infectious and very greatly appreciated.

Anne McIntyre of the Cotswold Healing Centre for her helpful suggestions.

And the many readers of the *Post and Echo* newspaper features for their interest and the fund of knowledge they shared with me. It's very encouraging to know that someone actually reads what you write!

Last, but not least, my wife Ann, who as guide, mentor, editor and adviser steered this book from an idea into a finished manuscript, translating the torrent of paper into a coherent whole; and our son Robin, who for the last year has shared his home with piles of manuscript.

Author's Note

This book deals with natural products of the countryside, woods and fields, and readers may be tempted into thinking that, because plant-based medicines come from a natural countryside source, they are harmless. This would be a dangerous assumption to make, for although I have attempted to avoid recommending herbal remedies compounded from toxic plants, misidentification of a plant in the field could lead to fatal consequences, and a number of common plants are lethal in quite small doses.

Use only those plants you know for certain are correctly identified and if you have even the slightest doubt consult someone who is experienced in herbal medicine. Or better still, obtain your supplies of herbs from a recognized herbalist or pharmacist.

It is unwise, if not downright dangerous, to treat yourself for anything other than the simplest ailments and injuries. Do maintain the strictest standards of hygiene with utensils and dressings. All herbal preparations such as infusions and compresses are best used *absolutely fresh*. Do not attempt to keep them.

Remember, too, that it is unlawful to treat other people unless you have a medical qualification which allows you to do so.

Lastly, your medical practitioner should be your ally in the search for good health and should be consulted before you commence any course of self-treatment with herbal medicine for any but the simplest common ills.

The laws that govern the practice of medicine in the United Kingdom are relatively liberal and anyone can sell herbs for medical purposes. However, herbal medicine is controlled by more regulations than other forms of alternative medicine. When the Medicines Act was brought in, in 1968, restrictions were put on a number of the more potentially poisonous herbs. So although there is no law to stop you from growing foxglove, mistletoe, or poison ivy in your garden for your own personal use, the Medicines Act forbids you to sell or prescribe them to anyone else, unless you are a qualified doctor or pharmacist.

Herbs that herbalists are not allowed to supply are as follows: areca, Canadian hemp, *Catha edulis, Chenopodium ambrosides, Cocculus indicus*, crotalaria, croton oil, croton seed, *Cucurbita maxima*, duboisia, elaterium, embelia, ergot, *Erysimum canescens*, holarrhena, ignatius bean, kamala, kousso, male fern, podophyllum, pomegranate bark, sabadilla, santonica, savin, scopolia, stavesacre seeds, stropanthus, slippery elm bark, veratrum and yohimbe bark.

Another group of herbs which are available from herbalists, but only in very limited dosages and with clearly written instructions, are: aconite, adonis, belladonna, celandine, cinchona, colchicum, conium, convallaria, ephedra, gelsemium, henbane, jaborandi, lobelia, poison oak, quebracho, ragwort, and thorn-apple.

In the course of writing this book I have gone to great lengths to ensure that the plants listed are non-toxic in their effect providing they are used in the proportions recommended. However, these proportions have been shown mainly in metric measures, although some are in teaspoonfuls or handfuls, which are universally understood.

To convert metric to imperial measurements the following guide may be valuable.

Dry measurement	Liquid measurement
28.4g = 1oz	122ml = $\frac{1}{4}$ pint
100g = $3\frac{1}{2}$oz	284ml = $\frac{1}{2}$ pint
500g = 1.1lb	568ml = 1 pint
1kilo = 2.2lb	1litre = $1\frac{3}{4}$ pints

However, it is obviously sensible to use round quantities! For instance, if I have suggested using 30g of plant to 1litre of water, then you could safely put 1oz in $1\frac{1}{2}$ pints of water to obtain the correct concentration of active ingredients in the finished brew.

Introduction

This book was born out of curiosity. My work as a naturalist and observer of the countryside – mainly birds and animals to begin with – brought me into contact with a host of plants which appeared to be connected, albeit sometimes rather tenuously, with the practice of herbal medicine.

For instance, why is marsh woundwort so called? Why should the Latin and Greek international scientific titles of some plants contain the word *officinalis*, indicating medicinal use in the past? My interest became further aroused when reading about the history of medicine generally. It's not too difficult to envisage primitive man (and I hesitate to call him this for our ancestors were more in tune with their environment than we of the twentieth century) stretching and rising stiffly to his feet after a disturbed night caused by a surfeit of woolly rhino meat or perhaps a tough piece of mammoth. Very likely his first action would be to wander off into the surrounding countryside to find a plant to relieve the spasms in his distended gut and calm his throbbing head. Having found what he was looking for, he would return to his waking family to dispense the soothing weed.

Even today, we in the developed Western world are much preoccupied with the state of our health. My initial attitude to the science of herbal medicine was one of scepticism. For a modern man in a modern country it seemed like casting the runes to contemplate the medicinal benefits of wild and not-so-wild plants. Yet the seed of curiosity was well and truly sown in my mind when it became increasingly obvious to me that certain plants had quite a variety of regional names and these particular plants were the ones that medieval herbalists had used most for their potions.

Bearing in mind the difficulty of communications between settlements in the early centuries of this millennium, and the rarity of anyone other than monks and priests who could read or write, there must have been sufficient real benefit from the use of certain plants to give the populace good reason to believe in their efficacy and to immortalize them with popular local names.

Even so, having noted relationships between the proliferation of regional names and the medicinal value of certain plants to medieval herbalists, I still found it difficult to consider herbal medicine as anything other than a fascinating historical study until I happened across a book containing a reference to the fact that before 1920 over 90% of all medicines listed in the *British Pharmacopoeia* were plant-based. Indeed, our dependence on plant-based medicaments was prevalent until well into the twentieth century.

As a naturalist I've always been deeply interested in all aspects of the countryside – birds, animals, insects and plants – but it was not until commissioned to write a series of weekly articles on medicinal plants called 'Health from the Hedgerow' for the *Hertfordshire and Bedfordshire Evening Post and Echo* that I really became immersed in the relationship of plants to the treatment of the diseases of man and animals.

There are many branches of what has become known as 'alternative medicine', from acupuncture to faith healing. I do not intend to venture into these rarified realms here, but will content myself with the properties of those plants and derivatives valued by the homoeopath, the herbalist and the conventional pharmacist.

I will attempt to avoid the use of obscure technical terms, for a practice does not become any more legitimate by surrounding itself with complex terminology. For instance, why say that the action of coltsfoot is 'anti-tussive' when all we need to know is that it relieves coughs?

It was only a few short years ago that the sophisticated westerner looked down on vegetarianism as if this were only one step away from the psychiatrist's couch. Now most high streets sport a well-stocked health food shop.

It is reasonable to say that generally the health standards of individuals interested in alternative medicine is better than the mass of the population, due to the fact that interest in homeopathy and herbalism usually goes hand-in-hand with a greater awareness of the body's need for a well-balanced healthy diet, rich in fibre and low in sodium salts and animal fats, and the necessity to keep both muscles and mind in good order by sensible regimes of exercise and relaxation.

The study of herbalism also helps people become more aware of the natural world of plants and animals with which we share this planet, bringing home the idea that a healthy environment for the naturally occurring denizens of the countryside is also a healthy environment for the human race – something we should all strive to achieve.

The first herbals were compiled in the reign of the Chinese Emperor Shen Nung and attributed to him *circa* 3000 BC. However, there is excellent reason to believe that the Emperor and his scribes were merely compiling a list of plants and remedies that had been in regular use in China for a thousand years before his reign and very likely a considerable time before that. The tradition is still carried on today in modern China with the famous 'barefoot doctor' service, which depends mainly on herbalism for many day-to-day cures for the peoples of that teeming nation.

China's medical skills were exported by spice and silk traders to the emerging western cultures via the pharoah-dominated lands of the Middle East and Egypt. Egypt itself was a repository for the Sumerian herbal tradition written down only a few years later than that of the Chinese. As with the Chinese, the Sumerians were merely recording information passed down to them from earlier civilizations and many of their regular constituents would be familiar to herbalists today.

Some of the things that make up our modern culture were codified by the Greeks: information not only about the therapeutic use of drugs derived from plants, but about the plants themselves and their propagation. The name of Hippocrates, a physician of the fifth century BC, is synonymous with medicine and doctors, through the Hippocratic oath. Although he didn't compile herbals himself, he practised medicine in a way that would find favour among many of today's advanced medical theorists: that of allowing the body's own defence mechanism to fight illness with just a little help from medicine.

Aristotle, a Greek philosopher who lived 384 to 322 BC, wrote about the properties of herbs and their propagation in his *De Somnia*, but it was Theophrastus who compiled a herbal called *His Enquiry into Plants*, which became the foundation of botanical texts for hundreds of years. His work on the classification of plants and their effect was continued in Rome by Pliny the Elder (AD 23 to AD 79) with his *Natural History*. Doubtless Pliny would have continued this work had not the volcano Vesuvius cut short his stay on earth by an untimely eruption.

The Greeks were physicians to the known world when Rome culturally was in the ascendant, and it was Dioscorides who, in the first century AD, codified medicinal plants from all over the world and their uses. He was a military doctor and widely travelled, and his work formed the basis for all major herbals until the reign of Elizabeth I of England.

The physician Galen, born in AD 130, also studied the effect of medicine, but unlike Hippocrates, who lived from 460 to 377 BC, considered that the body needed the aid of medicines if it was to combat ills. Like Dioscorides, Galen's work survived well into the second millennium. Unfortunately a clear, reasoned approach to medicine was clouded by the teachings of several misguided physicians, one of whom was Galen, and during the fifteenth and sixteenth centuries the 'Doctrine of Signatures' was propounded.

Briefly, this meant that if a plant resembled a particular part of the body then it should be used to treat maladies affecting this part. Thus were members of the orchis group of plants, with their tuberous paired roots, added to the list of aphrodisiacs because of their resemblance to the male testes.

However, it would be unfair to associate Galen only with a system of medicine that was, at best, tenuously connected to the actual power of plants. In his less fanciful moments he did study and popularize a system of correct dosages. He provided a set of guidelines for the prescription of drugs, whereas prior to that time there had been no standards laid down at all.

Herbal knowledge in the Middle Ages and in medieval Europe was the province of the Church, especially monasteries and convents. Many of the surgeon priests were highly skilled.

Though history does not list their names, we know that they researched the work of the Greeks and Romans and wrote knowledgeable texts, albeit in Latin, a language of which the population as a whole had little knowledge. It was not until the Elizabethan herbalists came on the scene that all this useful information became available in the English language.

John Gerard, who lived from 1545 to 1612 and practiced medicine in Holborn, London, gathered together the acquired know-how of the monks after the dissolution of the monasteries in Henry VIII's reign. He compiled a history of plants that inspired a succession of herbals, culminating in that of Nicholas Culpeper, still in print to this day.

Culpeper practised in London, apart from his service in the Civil War, and during his short life (he died aged only 38 years) wrote a vast treatise. However, the Doctrine of Signatures had a few remaining devotees, of whom Culpeper was one. His preoccupation seems to have been a marriage of medical herbalism with astrology, and consequently much of his valuable work is clouded with references to the zodiac. Even so, it's an interesting document and there are pearls of wisdom tucked away within its pages. His main service to the science of herbalism was to make the whole subject more accessible to a wider section of the public by means of the written word.

James I enjoyed the ministrations of the court apothecary John Parkinson (1567 to 1650), whose *Theatre of Plants* was a dissertation of far more accurate observations than Culpeper's herbal, owing a great deal more to the research of the Greeks and Romans than to astrology and mysticism.

The diaries of John Evelyn who, unlike Culpeper, lived a long life, being 86 years old when he died, are a window on to the world of the days when herbal medicine was enjoying its heyday. They are valuable for the concise, accurate observations made and show how small a part hygiene and preventative medicine played during the time of the great plagues which so devastated the populace, altering the economic basis of society as the working and artisan classes died in their thousands. Evelyn, who was a scholar, also wrote a book on the culture of trees called *Sylva*, and translated from the French on the subject of gardens and gardening in general.

The upheaval of the Civil War and the great plague of the mid-seventeenth century changed medical thinking somewhat and an interchange of ideas with the Continent, most particularly France, added more and more medicinal plants to the herbal armoury of the English physician. The French still place considerable reliance on herbs for medicinal use and this is regarded as an extension of conventional medicine rather than as an alternative. In most of western Europe pharmacists tend to sell preparations of herbs as part of their normal stock in trade, whereas their English counterparts rarely carry large stocks of herbal preparations, which are more usually purchased through health food stores or specialist herbal suppliers.

Research into the healing properties of plants is being carried on today all over the world, for there are thousands of trees and shrubs and lowly ferns whose properties have still to be investigated. Who knows – the magic bullet, the drug to cure all ills, the elixir of life for which the herbalist astrologers once strived may be growing quietly somewhere on the other side of the world!

What of modern herbal medicine and its practitioners? What is its relevance to modern man in a modern society?

The health of the Western nations rests largely on the provision of a clean water supply, an efficient sewage disposal system and a sufficiency of food. However, for some the very food they eat is their undoing. It is certainly strange that in a world where at least one-third of the population is starving one of the fastest growing industries among Western cultures is the provision of facilities for overweight people to rid themselves of excess fatty tissue. It is an alarming fact that in the West the largest killers are diseases connected with excessive consumption (be it of alcohol, tobacco or fatty foods), or cancers, caused in many cases by the way we live today.

Yet our health is still remarkable. In Europe and North America the twin evils of stark poverty and ignorance of hygiene have been almost eradicated, and it is these factors, even more than the effects of modern drugs, that are responsible for our healthy state and long lifespan.

Doses of potent modern drugs are prescribed by the thousand,

and increasingly there are cases where they are being given to patients to relieve some other drug-induced illness. This is probably something that has always happened; modern drugs are not alone in producing side-effects, some of them undesirable, but now it is happening on a larger scale with far more devastating repercussions.

Let me reassure you. This is not diatribe against modern drugs although as with all benefits to mankind, they can cause problems if misused. The purpose of this book is to give reliable, factual information about the known properties of certain plants, and those properties ascribed to them, and perhaps to speculate briefly on the potential of the thousands of species of plants in the secret wildernesses of the world; the rainforests, swamps and wetlands, mountains and oceans that may possibly hold the key to the degenerative diseases of a modern civilization.

After all, it was from the natives of the Amazon basin that the drug curare was discovered. Now it greatly assists many modern surgical procedures, particularly heart surgery, and the melon-like plant, the yam, that is thought to have supplied an early version of the drug contained in the modern contraceptive pill was found in a rainforest environment. We should pause and consider what we may lose before we wantonly destroy such a cornucopia.

From the very beginning, the practice of medicine has been rather like that of a secret society, and in some ways it is wise that it should be so. However, there have been occasions in history such as that in the reign of Henry VIII when the barber surgeons developed the 'closed shop' to such a degree that there was an act prohibiting the practice of herbal medicine. This was in force for some two years until the populace, unable to bear the cost of the state-protected medical service, forced the barber surgeons into allowing herbalists to ply their trade again.

Today there is a justified reluctance by the majority of Health Service doctors to embrace the gentler arts of herbalism. A modern GP's practice is typified by a full waiting room and a list of patients who are allowed little time to communicate with their busy doctor. Whereas in the past a harassed mother would have been allowed to unburden her soul to her doctor and then be sent away with a harmless 'tonic' to give her confidence in her ability to cope with day-to-day problems, now powerful drugs that modify behaviour patterns and suppress the symptoms of depression are issued like sweets to a fractious child. And the pharmaceutical industry has an income that would be envied by many of the smaller countries in the Third World.

Yet in the countryside there are plants growing at our feet that can and do relieve the symptoms of minor ills. Some of these plants may be toxic, but even these have value in the hands of a qualified medical herbalist. A good herbalist is someone who has passed through an intensive course organized by a recognized body such as the Institute of Medical Herbalists, founded in 1864. Members of this Institute and others like it believe in healing the body with remedies from natural sources. Of course, there are charlatans in the herbal business, just as you will find charlatans in any walk of life, especially where there is an opportunity to extract money from a frightened or gullible public. But there are several established organizations who list recognized practitioners in this field, and you will find them on pages 201–3.

Certain serious illnesses require treatment under the aegis of the conventional health service and it would not be sensible to attempt to treat any but the most minor ailments without knowledge of the underlying cause of illness.

Wherever practicable, the advice of a properly qualified person should be sought when collecting herbs and wild plants, and you will need to be careful to pick only those that are not protected by any act or statute. All in all, it's a good idea to cultivate a clean, uncontaminated supply of herbal products in your own garden. Many of the more tender and exotic plants can be grown in a greenhouse with the minimum of effort and expense, and details of cultivation and preparation can be found on pages 184–7.

Those plants covered by the Wildlife and Countryside Act are listed on page 203ff., together with a list of other plants which are protected in the United States.

The North American Indians are a prime example of a people compatible with nature. They accrued a vast reservoir of herbal knowledge, yet in Western society we consider that our ancestors opened up the benefits of civilization to these peoples, who in fact had previously lived in complete harmony with and total dependence on the natural products of that vast continent. When the Pilgrim Fathers ventured across the Atlantic they complained of virtual starvation, whilst the native population lived well off the products of the land.

There are still a few isolated races whose dependence on their surroundings for the necessities of daily life is as real today as it was when our ancestors daubed themselves with a plant extract called woad to make them fearless and also to protect their skin from wound infections, woad being an antiseptic. The Bushmen of the Kalahari can put on weight and thrive in a landscape where a European would die of thirst and hunger in a week, to say nothing of the problems of heatstroke. Sadly, Bushman culture is vanishing with progress and we shall lose their simple wisdom which is passed on by word of mouth.

We are fortunate in that we have the benefit of the written word, but there must be many people, especially senior citizens, who retain in some corner of their mind invaluable folklore which has not yet been written down. It could be that some of them have herbal skills of great significance to the twentieth century.

The Herbs

Aaron's rod

(Verbascum thapsus)
Family: SCROPHULARIACEAE

USA: Aaron's rod, flannel plant, garden mullein, great mullein, mullein dock, velvet plant

Common in the English country-side before the agricultural revolution of the 1960s when the majority of traditional meadows and wood-land margins came under intensive cultivation, this tall native of damp meadowland and chalk pasture is also known as mullein, and in days gone by when far greater reliance was placed on plants, the fluff-covered leaves also earned it the name of 'blanket weed'. This may derive from the fact that the peasantry of the Middle Ages put the furry leaves in their crude leather shoes as insoles.

The history of Aaron's rod is long and illustrious. Its name is thought to have come about because of a likeness in the tall flowering spike to the staff of Levi which had Aaron's name inscribed upon it. When the rod was struck into the ground the upper part miraculously flowered. This plant seems to bloom in just such a miraculous way, a seemingly random blossoming over the flower spike consisting of tightly packed buds and seed capsules.

Romans employed the furry covering as wicks for oil lamps and the stems, too, were made into torches after being dried and dipped in tallow. They were an excellent lightweight source of illumination.

The grey fur protects the plant against insect attack and tends to prevent dessication of the large leaves by providing a layer of insulation against the drying effects of sun and wind.

This plant's medicinal virtues are known on both sides of the Atlantic, and American Indians smoke its leaves as a tobacco to relieve bronchial troubles, though this is not to be recommended since taking smoke into already inflamed bronchial tubes and throats is bound to cause more problems than it might be supposed to cure.

Mullein was better known in Britain for treating cattle, a rare tribute, for a peasant's cattle were his wealth and any medicine used on his treasured cows or oxen must have been well proven before it would be contemplated.

The increase in pulmonary tuberculosis brought about by a shift in population, in the nineteenth century, with farm workers and peasants moving into towns with unhealthy atmospheres and working conditions, brought Aaron's rod renewed medical popularity. It was found to be valuable for relieving early symptoms of this disease, although it could have had little effect on the cause, as lung damage progressed to its almost inevitable conclusion.

Notwithstanding this, a brew of the leaves and flowers together with honey, nutmeg and other spices was very popular not only for chest infections, but for sore gums and inflamed throats, and it is still prescribed as a gargle today.

This particular remedy has been recommended for hay fever and also to be applied externally to swollen glands, infections and inflammations, where its use as a fomentation bound to a swollen area with a piece of cloth was said to reduce swelling.

Culpeper recommended Aaron's rod for treating bleeding piles and bowel infections, but the value of the plant in such cases is now in some doubt, as these symptoms may be caused by an illness far more serious than simple inflammation and should be investigated by a qualified person.

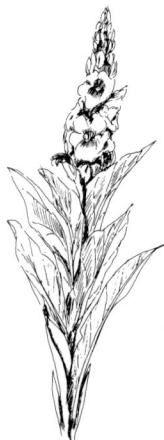

In the past, dried flowers were used as a sedative for children and as a gentle cure for headaches and fevers, but care should be taken with their storage as they will discolour rapidly if exposed to light. A cupful of dried flowers may be steeped in 1 litre of water for 10 minutes then strained. Drink as required. This was also said to be a remedy for warts and skin eruptions; in fact, a general cure-all.

Absinthe
(Artemisia absinthium)
Family : COMPOSITAE

USA : common wormwood

Otherwise known as wormwood,

this common garden plant is a native of Europe and sometimes found in waste places or on uncultivated ground.

It's a small shrub with silvery-grey foliage and slightly downy leaves and stems, and in summer its tiny yellow pompom-shaped flowers cover the tips of the growing points. It grows quite tall, reaching a metre in height, and bushes out from a series of thick woody stems.

It's hard to imagine that this attractive herb, demurely growing in suburban gardens, was once the subject of social upheaval, for it was from an extract of this plant that the drink absinthe was prepared. Compounded with alcohol, absinthe caused havoc in France throughout all social classes and aroused as much disquiet in the late nineteenth and early twentieth centuries as the use of dangerous drugs does in our own time.

In 1915 the French government prohibited its manufacture because it had brought about a new form of addiction and coupled with the high level of alcoholism already prevalent in France was becoming a serious health hazard.

Excessive drinking of absinthe caused a marked deterioration among addicts, inducing epilepsy and delusions of increasing frequency and terror leading to mental decline and eventual insanity. It is still used today, but only as a flavouring to the popular aperitif vermouth.

In concentration an extract of

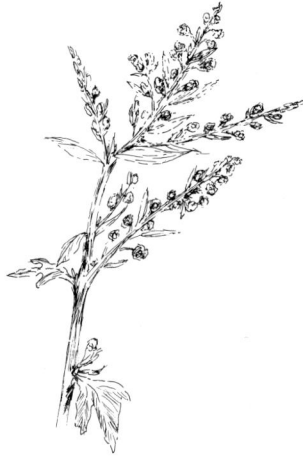

the plant is poisonous, but in small quantities it can be exceedingly useful as an aid to digestion and over a limited period of time is valuable for treating a number of simple ills and toning up the nervous system.

The Greeks valued its properties and Galen recommended it for worms and also to promote menstrual discharge. Consequently it is not a herb to be used in the early stages of pregnancy, or indeed during any part of pregnancy. *All* preparations that have a reputation for promoting menstruation or regularizing the menstrual cycle should be avoided during pregnancy.

The name wormwood, used in some country districts, comes directly from its reputation as a preparation for killing intestinal parasites and worms. For thread worms an old recipe advocates steeping 30g of fresh-pounded plant in a litre of beer for 4 days. This is strained, and 1 wineglass per day at breakfast time for no longer than 4 days is the recommended dose.

It's a pity that this herb, which was mentioned in the Bible and reputedly worn by John the Baptist as a girdle, has fallen into disrepute. The Greeks ascribed its virtues to the goddess Artemis and it was used by herbalists in the distant past in Mediterranean countries as a symbol of healing.

The pungency of the crushed leaves and stems is valuable in places where mosquitoes and midges are a nuisance, for the bitter oils make an effective deterrent, and a lotion made from 30g of crushed leaves and flowers added to 1 litre of boiling water is a long-established treatment for fleas and lice.

Incidentally, there is an unproven theory that this same infusion will reduce loss of hair if rubbed into the scalp night and morning.

Ancient herbals recommend absinthe as a cure for dysentery and for reducing the pain caused by gastric upset. This could well stem from its properties as a depressant and anti-parasitic, enabling the weakened alimentary tract to recover more quickly from illness.

Although there are distinct side effects to be considered when using absinthe, especially in high concentration, when employed as directed by a qualified herbalist it can be safe and beneficial.

Acacia
(Acacia vera, Acacia senegal)
Family: LEGUMINOSAE

The most famous of all the products obtained from this widely spread family of trees are water soluble resins known collectively as 'gum arabic', and the individual tree best known for its production of the beads of resin collected as they ooze naturally from the bark is the gnarled and twisted *Acacia senegal* (pictured).

In order for production to be increased, the trees are encouraged to exude more resin by cutting the bark with a sharp knife.

Gum arabic has been used for many years as a lubricant for the mucous membranes, for it combines readily with water to form a gel and in dilution also acts as a perfect medium for the finely dispersed pigments in artist's watercolours.

Medicinally it has been known for hundreds of years, and there is little doubt that gum from acacia trees was used by Egyptians at the time of the Pharoahs as a treatment for throat infections and as a constituent in other herbal remedies. A gum derived from the Egyptian thorn, *Acacia vera*, was very popular in the latter part of Queen Victoria's reign, being prescribed as acacia balsam. This was a highly praised cure-all whose uses ranged from a calming agent for the stomach to a treatment for gonorrhoea.

However, it would seem that its

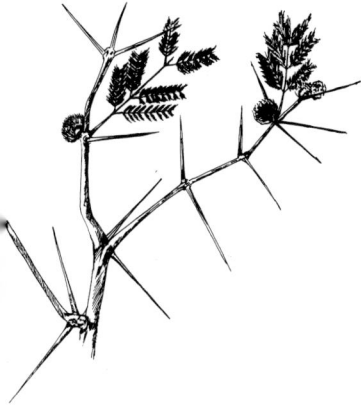

of Signatures, who ascribed many virtues to it. It is actually a fern, but the leaf has the look of a serpent's tongue. This being so, it's surprising that the medieval herbalist didn't put it at the top of the list for treating bites caused by venomous beasts.

However, the likelihood of finding an adder lurking where this plant grows is not great, for its favourite habitat is old meadowland, especially where it is damp, and this is just the sort of place adders avoid.

The simple green leaf has at its base a hard spike growing from the common stem. It is a small plant, easily overlooked, for although quite common in southern England it is not generally noted by country ramblers or walkers.

During the renaissance of herbalism in the seventeenth century it was a common herb for wound healing. Heat 30g of adder's tongue in a $\frac{1}{4}$ litre of olive oil for about an hour; the oil must not be allowed to boil. When cool, strain off the oil

greatest benefit was in treating throat infections, where it was used as a powder dissolved in water and in conjunction with other agents such as thymol. Moreover, it has virtues as a gentle laxative, was thought of as being very good for the relief of chest infections and was considered an excellent dietary supplement for consumptives, since it was kind to the digestion.

Though still used in food preparation, it is now more widely employed in the paint-making and printing industry as a pigment dispersal agent.

Adder's tongue
(Ophioglossum vulgatum)
Family: OPHIOGLOSSACEAE

A strange plant, this one, and it's easy to see why it was regarded with some awe by early herbalists, especially devotees of the Doctrine

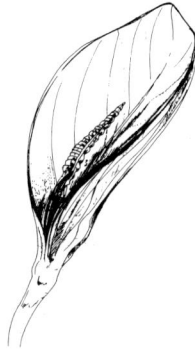

and use to treat open cuts and infected sores and grazes. This recipe was recommended in some herbals as a remedy for infected varicose leg ulcers.

Another of its uses was for treating chilblains, when oil or an ointment prepared by pounding a teaspoon of chopped adder's tongue into an equal amount of commercial cold cream was applied to an affected area. This is still valid today. Being cold and therefore unsterilized, this cream must be used fresh, as it will keep for only a few days. The oil or prepared cream should be spread on a clean piece of lint and placed over chilblains with a bandage, or alternatively spread on a piece of adder's tongue leaf bound over the chilblains with a bandage. This is a very old remedy used by the Romanies.

Agrimony
(Agrimonia eupatoria)
Family: ROSACEAE

USA: stickweed, tall agrimony

High summer in the English countryside would not be complete without agrimony. The tall star-flowered spike reaches above the meadow grasses as if deliberately seeking the sun.

The name agrimony would appear to be a misnomer, being a corruption of a Greek mistranslation from medieval times. Apparently during translation of

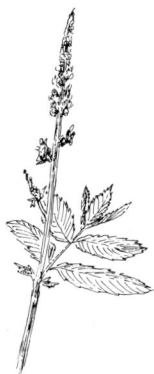

Pliny's writings the name of a small crop weed poppy (*Papaver argemone*) common in Mediterranean countries was mistakenly applied to agrimony. It seems the original poppy was used to treat eye disorders, especially a white spot on the cornea, but there is no record of agrimony ever being used to treat eye problems.

The greatest benefit to the eye from this attractive plant is its pleasing appearance. It is a member of the family rosaceae, and the small brilliant yellow flowers are typically star-shaped.

Although it grows in many waste places, it prefers a chalky habitat and preferably relic chalk downland. It will grow along meadowland margins where no herbicide spray or fertilizer has been used, and it can be grown from seed, but it is difficult to get it started.

It flowers in the latter part of July and early August, and should be gathered before the petals fully open and dried in the shade in an airy place at a temperature no higher than 38° centigrade (100° Fahrenheit).

Agrimony has been used since the Middle Ages for cuts and grazes, as it has a slightly antiseptic effect and the tannin content is astringent and stems bleeding; the volatile oils contained in the leaves and flowers are anti-inflammatory too.

In modern times the active principles of agrimony have been prescribed to treat gastric upsets, and it is often used as a general tonic for the digestive tract. The French have several good recipes for a tonic tea made from the dried leaves. It is a reddish colour, and though astringent and slightly bitter, it's very popular.

The constituents of agrimony are soluble in water and the method of preparing a brew of leaves and flowers, to be taken either internally or externally, is as follows: 5g of dried leaves and flowers infused in $\frac{1}{4}$ litre of boiling water for 20 minutes and if necessary flavoured with a little honey. It can be taken as a mouthwash for gum irritations and sore throats. Public speakers and singers might take a special note here, as this infusion is said to be very beneficial when used as a gargle. Unsweetened, it is widely recommended for cystitis.

It has been administered as a remedy for jaundice, but its properties might be considered by some to be too mild to have much value in treating this illness, or for the morbid watery accumulation known as dropsy.

On the Continent they have another method of preparing agrimony for external use, for both humans and animals: 200g of dried leaves and flowers are boiled in a litre of red wine for 5 minutes, left to stand for 1 hour, and strained. The tepid brew is applied to wounds that are slow to heal, such as varicose ulcers, and also in a compress for sprains.

This plant has as many uses as it has flowers on its spike, for as well as medicinal properties the flowers yield a yellow dye that deepens in shade in the fullness of summer.

Alder

(Alnus glutinosa)
Family: BETULACEAE

Wherever you find alder trees there is little doubt you are close to water, be it above or below ground level, for this is a tree that relishes damp places.

Left untended, alders will grow into mighty trees of over 20m (66ft). They are quite common over much of the northern hemisphere and closely related to American red alders (*Alnus rubra*) or Oregon alders. The American variety has saw-edged leaves, but its medicinal virtues are similar to the British tree.

The common alder has been much cultivated in the United

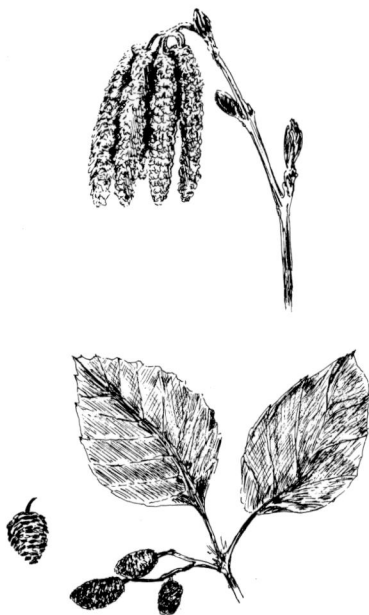

Kingdom, where it loves the damp climate. Its timber has been used for brush backs and for fencing stakes in marshy areas, for the timber is water-resistant. Until the advent of smokeless gunpowder in the latter half of the nineteenth century, alders were grown in coppice stands to produce poles suitable for charcoal for the gunpowder industry. It was thought that alder charcoal was the finest for this purpose.

In consequence of this coppicing and subsequent neglect of woodlands where the coppice stools have matured into major trees, a great many of the alders we see today are in poor condition and often at the end of their lives. They grow easily from root propagation, and where regeneration has been allowed to continue the familiar shape of this attractive tree graces river banks and valley bottoms.

They were exported to the Americas with the first settlers as medicinal stock and probably also for the charcoal potential of the mature plant. However, American Indians, possessors of a long history of association with the red alder that grows in a similar habitat, were already familiar with an infusion of the inner bark to ease mouth and throat infections.

There is a noteworthy parallel in the fact that both American Indians and English farmworkers put alder leaves in their shoes to keep their feet comfortable and cool.

The name 'alder' goes back to Anglo-Saxon times, for even then it was prized. It was used mainly to treat gangrene, a common occurrence following wounds caused by battle axes and war clubs where tissues were pulverized by the force of the blow. The anti-inflammatory value of alder is well documented, and one method of applying it to reduce pain and swelling from bruises is to pound the leaves into a poultice with a little milk and bind to the swelling.

There are also references in some old herbals to the use of alder for relieving breast congestion and mastitis.

The dried bark, usually already ground to a powder, is available from most herbalists. It is astringent and often prescribed in the company of other herbs or with a little honey, especially where it is being used for sore throats. Half a teaspoon of alder bark, a tablespoon of dried wild marjoram and honey to taste infused in $\frac{1}{2}$ litre of boiling water for 10 minutes and used as a gargle can prove very comforting indeed.

Its scientific suffix, *glutinosa*, refers to the gluey texture of the crushed leaves. They should be gathered when young and fresh and dried very quickly in an airing cupboard on a muslin screen, then stored in dark glass airtight jars to keep the colour and active ingredients intact.

Alder buckthorn

(Frangula alnus)
Family: RHAMNACEAE

Despite its name, alder buckthorn is not related to the alder, being a member of quite a different family of plants. It grows in damp marshy habitats in south-east England and a near relative is common buckthorn, also used medicinally.

Herbalists usually dry and store the bark (the most useful part of the plant) for a period of time in order to modify some of the active ingredients. It should not be used fresh, as it is a powerful purgative that can cause severe irritation of the large intestine and it should not be taken in any but the smallest quantities.

It is advisable to obtain it at herbalists', where it is available as a tincture or in syrup, and to use only under medically qualified direction.

For medicinal purposes, bark taken from the twigs is best. It should be dried very quickly in the sun then stored loose in a dark place, not sealed in a jar or packet, until it has aged.

Dry skin can sometimes benefit from a lotion made from alder buckthorn bark. Steep 100g of bark in 1 litre of boiling water, allow to cool, then apply either as a lotion or compress.

The twigs can be prepared as fine drawing or medicinal charcoal, being straight and hard, and like common alder, the charcoal obtained from alder buckthorn twigs was also employed to

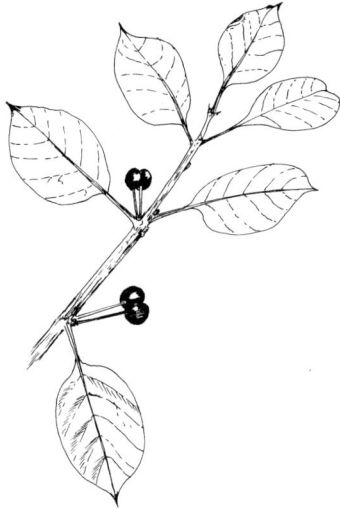

preparing a fine sporting gun-powder.

Alder buckthorn's long straight twigs were also once used for cane seating and basketwork, together with willow or split alder.

Alfalfa/Sweet lucerne

(Medicago sativa)
Family: LEGUMINOSAE

When Nature designed her grand plan she surely singled out the pea family for the benefit of man, or so it would seem. Until recently the whole efficacy of the fallow agriculture and crop rotational sys-tem of the countryside hung on the ability of legumes to fix free nitro-gen in the soil and make it available to other plants. This miracle comes about by the action of a bacterium residing in the root nodules of leguminous plants.

During the Iron Age our distant ancestors thrived on the early cult-ivated beans they grew, and as these beans developed so they en-riched the very earth in which they rooted, allowing other more demanding crops to be sown with success; thereby hangs the history of agricultural settlement.

Clovers constitute another branch of this illustrious family, but traditionally they have always been fed to animals. Though they may not have the charisma of a *petit pois*, they are, none the less, even better for our bodies.

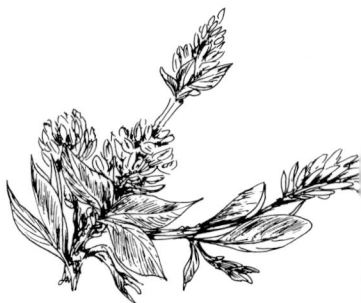

In America alfalfa is known as 'buffalo herb', but this rather dubious name hasn't prevented us from processing it into food for man, thereby bypassing the buf-falo completely.

A baby food known in America as Pabulum is prepared from the dried plant ground into a flour; it is ideally rich in protein and many easily assimilated minerals and trace elements. It is also a source of anti-haemorrhagic vitamin K, as well as vitamins A and D. Its use by country people in the United States for peptic ulcers has led to some rather more scientific investiga-tions being carried out into its possibilities as a food for patients suffering with stomach ulcers, and so far this research appears to bear out the positive results obtained by country herbalists.

Alfalfa, or lucerne, as it is known, grows best in the south of England and West Country, and if you want a fresh daily supply it grows freely from seed in the gar-den. Where it is grown for cattle feed there is always a possibility of contamination from sprays.

Fresh leaves can be added with other leaf salad vegetables as part of a mixed salad, and a handful of fresh growing shoots make a pleasant addition to sandwiches. The crushed dried plant can be made into a tea with mint leaves, as popularized in America, by infusing alfalfa and spearmint leaves together. Chill in a refrigerator and serve with honey, orange and lemon peel and peppermint leaf.

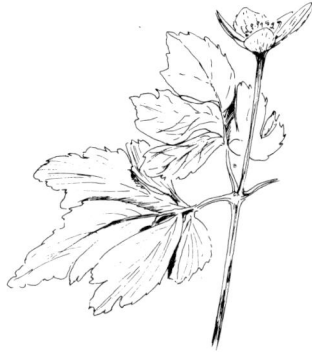

Anemone

(Anemone pulsatilla,
Anemone hepatica,
Anemone nemorosa)
Family: RANUNCULACEAE

Anemones come from one of those families of plants that man has adopted and adapted for both his garden and his medicine chest. The garden species are variable in colour and bloom in late winter when all other flowers are prudently hiding their heads, but the most widely used members of the family are the wild varieties: pasque flower (*Anemone pulsatilla*), wood anemone (*Anemone nemorosa*) (pictured), and common liverwort (*Anemone hepatica*).

Pasque flowers are one of the better-known medicinal anemones, even though the fresh leaves contain a poison similar to that found in aconite. Despite this problem they were traditionally employed as a treatment for nervous exhaustion and irritability,

and considered especially efficacious for blue-eyed, fair-haired women, who were thought to be more drastically affected by the upsets of the menstrual cycle.

Normally the root is not employed medicinally and use of the fresh plant is discouraged because it is extremely irritant in action. However, this property lessens considerably upon drying. Nowadays the use of pasque flower is limited to an alcoholic tincture for relieving menstrual pain.

The name 'pasque flower' derives from the fact that it usually blooms at Easter time. It was given its name when the Gregorian calendar was in use and Easter fell several weeks later than it does today. In consequence, the possibility of finding this strange, hairy blue bloom open on Easter day depends on the vagaries of the weather.

It would appear that of all the early-flowering anemones pasque flower is the earliest. A native of undisturbed chalk pastures, it is now very rare in England, appearing only on the Chiltern and Sussex Downs in protected sites.

One of the most attractive woodland plants is the wood anemone, otherwise known as the windflower on account of its strange habit of never opening its petals unless the wind is blowing. The flower of this attractive species is usually purest white, but very occasionally you will find pink tinges in the linen-like petals.

The juice of wood anemone used to be recommended to dispel phlegmatic humours and lethargy. It was supposed to be sniffed up the nostrils, and the results must have been quite dramatic, as it is an irritant and would have resulted in sneezing and gasping. Chewing the root was also recommended, for it was thought that spitting was a good way of ridding the body of poisons.

As well as being irritant, the juice is poisonous, and was often administered in large doses to people who were paralysed, with fatal results. It was supposed to cure them!

More often, though, the leaves or whole plant were boiled in water and the resulting brew used to clean and disinfect ulcers. An ointment was made by adding the juice of wood anemone to hog's grease. This was spread on sores and open festering wounds.

In America at the turn of the eighteenth century a solution of anemone was used to treat all manner of external injuries from scalds to syphilis, but these days little reliance is placed on remedies containing wood anemone because one of its constituents is unstable and can occur in toxic quantities in the prepared herb.

Less well known both as a plant and a medicinal herb is liverwort. This plant owes much of its popularity to the Doctrine of Signatures, which preached that any remedy for a particular part of the body was best found by using plants with flowers, leaves or roots resembling specific organs. The name *hepatica*, from the Latin *hepaticus* (of the liver) reflects this belief. In consequence, the fleshy liver-shaped leaves of hepatica were considered a sovereign remedy for illnesses of that organ.

Angelica
*(Angelica archangelica,
Angelica officinalis)*
Family: UMBELLIFEREAE

This plant was favoured as a treatment during the great plagues of the thirteenth and fourteenth centuries, when many hundreds of doses of angelica root were taken by a desperate populace to ward off the sickness. The flavour is such that repeated doses are extremely pleasant, being derived from the aromatic coumarin.

Like many popular herbs, it has several names, among them 'holy ghost' or 'root of the holy ghost'. It is thought this name came about because of the faith placed in its healing powers during the Milan plague of the early sixteenth century, although other chroniclers ascribe it to the fact that the plant often comes into flower on St Michael the Archangel's day, 8 May.

In common with other plants which were given holy significance, angelica was used in charms against witches and the evil eye. It is hard for us nowadays to imagine the awe in which the healing properties of this herb were held.

In Europe and the British Isles angelica is now used primarily as a candied cake decoration. Its bright-green glassy appearance certainly adds attraction to cakes and buns, yet in sixteenth-century London the candied stems were thought to be a potent medicine to ward off all manner of ills.

It is a plant of wet places and resembles common hedgeside cow parsley, being a member of the same family. Although it was introduced to this country as a garden plant, it can be found sometimes in damp river valleys or growing in marshy field corners.

It is important not to confuse it with another more dangerous plant called hemlock which belongs to the same family. Hemlock tends to be a smaller plant and has mottled reddish stems whereas angelica is tall, up to 2m in height, and the thick bright-green stems are deeply ridged, rather like the surface of celery.

A good general tonic and a calming agent for the stomach can be prepared from 20g of chopped root or alternatively 15g of crushed seeds, brought to the boil in 1 litre of water. Allow to cool for 1 hour. It is a stimulant and not recommended just before retiring to bed, and must not be taken in excessive quantities as it could cause paralysis of the central nervous system.

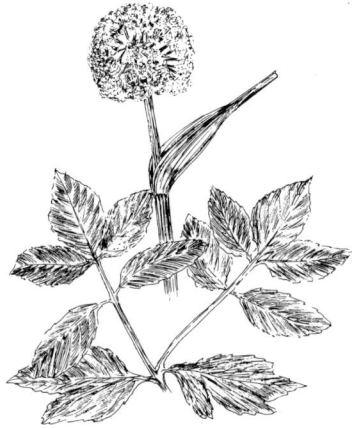

There are a number of records through the centuries of angelica being used to relieve migraine, vertigo and faintness. Quite a difference from the times when angelica was a principal ingredient in an elixir thought to prolong life, cure the bite of rabid dogs, heal ulcers, improve vision and also, when dropped into the ears, improve hearing.

Aniseed
(Pimpinella anisum)
Family: UMBELLIFERAE

The flavour of aniseed has always

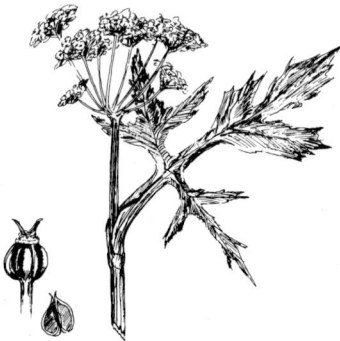

held great appeal for the human race and there are many plants that possess this flavour to a greater or lesser degree. However, the original plant from which the strong pungent oil was derived is anise.

Seeds of anise are used in confectionery. They are the crunchy bits in the middle of aniseed balls, although this sweet seems to have fallen from favour lately.

The strongly scented oil which is extracted from the seed is said to be almost a narcotic to dogs, and they certainly seem to find the smell very much to their liking. Trails laid with a trace of aniseed oil can be followed by a dog with only a moderately sensitive nose.

The remedies in which it was most popular were those connected with ailments of the digestive tract and for treating colic in small babies. Gripe water containing anise is still widely used today.

However, it is in the culinary field that aniseed has its greatest following. On the Continent seeds of anise are added to breads and cakes to impart a little piquancy to the finished article.

The use of anise in heavy cereal-based confections, often highly indigestible by themselves, is soundly based, for the aniseed flavour appears to promote saliva, so helping to begin the process of converting starch to a form more easily assimilated by the digestive system.

Aquilegia
(Aquilegia vulgaris)
Family: RANUNCULACEAE

It is unusual to find aquilegia in the wild in the British Isles, as its habitat of limestone pavement or hard chalk hills has been altered by quarrying and changes in agricultural practice. Where it does occur it is usually a garden escapee.

Its name derives from the shape of the nectar tubes of the ornate blue-white or lilac-pink flowers, which resemble the claws of a bird of prey. *Aquila* is the Latin name for an eagle, hence aquilegia.

Gerard talks of the plant as 'delighting the lion', and though he does not elaborate further there is good reason to believe that he was referring to the likeness of the claw-shaped flowers to a lion's paw.

Aquilegia's other name of columbine is again thought to be a reference to the shape of the flowers, comparing them to the form of doves or pigeons. The plant

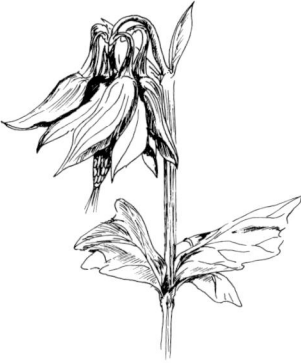

also has an Anglo-Saxon name, culvertwort, from *culfre*, the Anglo-Saxon word for pigeon.

It is obvious that this herb has a long history of association with man, and closer investigation reveals that it was used by herbalists of old for a variety of purposes, one of which appears to have been to procure abortions. References are made to the properties of columbine to speed childbirth, often a veiled allusion to abortion, which was both illegal and a mortal sin.

There are many references to columbine in the literature of the Middle Ages, and Shakespeare too often writes about the flower. In *Hamlet*, fennel and columbine are mentioned in tandem, the symbolism being fennel for flattery and columbine for ingratitude, as by Shakespeare's time columbine was the emblem for thankless lovers — perhaps another veiled reference to its use in abortion following an unsuccessful love affair.

In such cases the root is known to produce a toxic substance likely to kill the mother as well as the unborn child, and it seems that its use in hastening labour fell from favour early in medieval times, although it was still prescribed for sore throats, with fresh leaves prepared in boiling water as a gargle. However, the bitter taste must have deterred all but the strongest-spirited.

The seeds of aquilegia found favour for relieving urinary tract problems in the time of the Stuarts, a dram of the crushed seeds being administered in wine. This remedy was still used in France in the eighteenth century and even later as a specific for measles.

Nowadays aquilegia is found not in the herbalist's armoury, but gracing suburban gardens. Once established it is self-seeding and will flower year after year. However, if you have young children take extra care as it is poisonous.

Arnica
(Arnica montana)
Family: COMPOSITAE

One of the most useful plants in the herbal armoury is arnica. This plant similar to marigold is not a native of Great Britain but found in the more hilly and mountainous parts of Europe.

For many years, in the early history of herbal medicine, arnica found favour as a salve for treating bruises and as such is still in regular use today.

Arnica montana has a reputation for being toxic in large doses and because of this it has fallen from favour. The leaves and stem are covered with fine hook-like hairs that can cling to the inside of the mouth and throat lining, possibly causing attacks of nausea; but an extract of stem and flowers, properly strained and prepared, will cause far less irritation. However, the plant does contain a volatile oil which is best avoided, and there are far better herbal remedies for renal colic, one of the illnesses for which tincture of arnica used to be employed.

Nevertheless, a compress of fresh leaves and flowers is considered invaluable for bruises and minor cuts. The dried plant can be prepared as a tincture by soaking 100g of dried flowers in $\frac{1}{2}$ litre of alcohol. Only use pure alcohol from a chemist or alternatively a strong spirit such as vodka or aquavit. The dried flowers are the the most popular part of this herb, but if you are collecting plants from the wild (incidentally, it is protected in Switzerland where it grows sparsely) the whole plant can be dried and used for tinctures.

The tincture itself is rather powerful in its effect and should be used sparingly, never neat. It should be diluted, 1 tablespoon to $\frac{1}{2}$ litre of water for mild bruises and 1 tablespoon to $\frac{1}{4}$ litre of hot water for a hot compress for bad bruising or sprains.

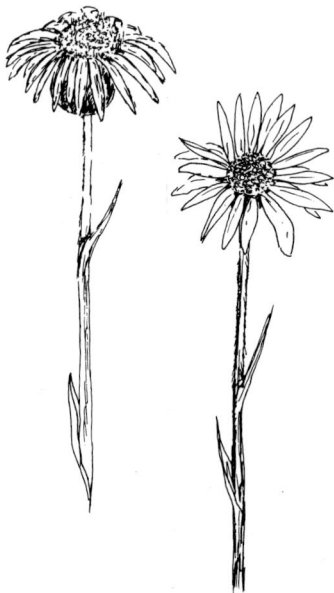

You may find that preparation of tinctures is too time-consuming or expensive, in which case an infusion of 15g of dried flowers to 1 litre of hot water or heated beer will give a satisfactory level of active ingredients. The alcohol in beer dissolves the volatile oils and other active principles better than water alone. A light bitter beer is best. As an added benefit, this brew will also contain the extracted principles of hops.

As mentioned earlier, arnica is an alpine plant found in the mountainous areas of Europe, on hillside pastures and screes up to 2,500m above sea level, growing best between 1000m and 2000m. It is tall and striking at 600cm with bright-yellow daisy-like flowers borne on long downy stems. The leaves, which are also downy and narrow grow alternately on the stem.

Because it is increasingly rare in its native habitat it's best to grow it from seed, picking the flowers when they open in July or August. Separate the petals from the flower heads by removing the green involucre at the base. The florets and petals should then be dried in an airing cupboard as quickly as possible and stored in tightly sealed dark-glass jars together with a dessicant cell to keep the moisture level as low as possible. This should keep for as long as the jar remains unopened.

Two drops of this tincture added to a little cold cream and mixed thoroughly should reduce the inflammation caused by those sore skin eruptions called blind boils.

Ash, common

(Fraxinus excelsior)
Family: OLEACEAE

Ash is a common tree in many parts of Europe, especially in the British Isles where the trees congregate in woodlands on chalk soil. For such a large tree, often over 30m (90ft) tall, it grows surprisingly quickly, and the seeds or ash keys germinate freely where they fall. In some areas they are so common as to be regarded almost as weeds.

However, in the days of Druids and Vikings and the old religions,

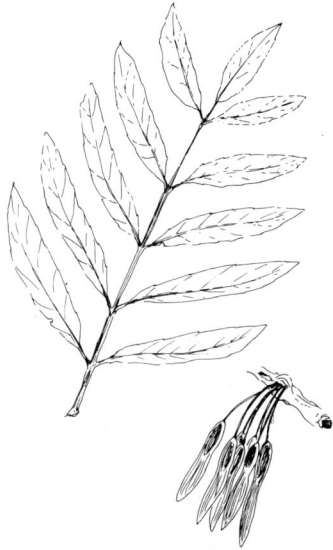

ash groves were temples where rites of spring and sacrifices of slaves and captives of war were carried out to appease the gods.

The Teutons especially revered ash trees, dedicating them to the god Thor. They used the straight-grained tough springy timber for the shafts of their spears, which they believed would always fly true and kill their enemies. The Greeks, too, considered that an ash spear-shaft would render them invincible. Legend has it that the great spear carried by Achilles was shafted in ash.

Once a tree begins to collect legends they soon multiply, and carrying an ash leaf shaped like the blade of a spear was considered to render the bearer immune from snakebite. This was a fairly safe legend to propagate, for there are very few cases of snakebite in Europe and the incidence of venomous snakes even in Greece is small.

The ash tree has considerable medicinal properties. Bark, leaves and ash seeds have all been found extremely useful. In the Middle Ages bark gathered in spring from small ash twigs and dried in the shade at a low temperature was ground and infused in water to reduce a patient's temperature and as a treatment for dropsy. It preceded quinine for alleviating malarial fevers, prescribed as a powder mixed with honey.

Ash was also known as the gout tree, for the leaves (more potent dried than fresh) become diuretic when infused in water. Leaves should be gathered in May and June and dried in a dark, warm, airy place, then kept in tightly sealed containers until required.

For relieving gout, 30g of the dried leaves infused in 1 litre of boiling water for 15 minutes and sometimes flavoured with mint can be taken 1 cupful at a time before meals, 3 times a day. This remedy has also been used in Europe and southern England for rheumatism.

It is said that if an infusion of ash leaves is taken every four weeks it will improve general health, and there are many recipes for ash tonics that have been praised for prolonging active life.

The Greeks considered that ash keys boiled in water were a mild aphrodisiac and a home-made alcoholic drink called frênette is prepared by steeping ash leaves, sugar and chicory with tartaric acid in hot water. When cool add yeast and allow to ferment. This is used as a tonic mainly in French country districts and also doubles as a gentle laxative.

Asparagus
(Asparagus officinalis)
Family: LILIACEAE

Mention to most people that asparagus is a medicinal plant and you will be given a variety of looks ranging from the slightly quizzical to the frankly disbelieving. However, it is quite true, for this tasty vegetable was indeed a well-known treatment for kidney, uri-

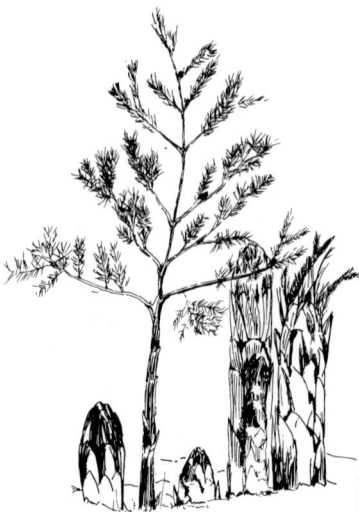

nary tract, and gall bladder infections, and was also a powerful diuretic used in the early days of medicine for water retention and dropsy.

If old herbals are to be believed, then infections of the urinary tract and various stones of the kidney and bladder used to be extremely commonplace. It may be, however, that there were considerable faults in the diagnosis of such illnesses.

The vicissitudes of life in the fifteenth and sixteenth centuries led to premature ageing and it was rare for an adult male to reach forty without falling prey to one of many ills as a result of poor diet and insufficient sanitation.

A species of asparagus (*Asparagus prostratus*) is a native of the United Kingdom, but it's a very rare plant confined to the softer climate of Devon, Dorset and the other counties of the west, and also south-east Ireland. It grows on sea cliffs facing the sun and in warm grassy places.

The asparagus familiar to us as a culinary delicacy is an import from the Mediterranean and grows wild in Israel, springing up after the rains, and although the finely divided leaflets of the fan-shaped foliage make the plant look like a fern, it is in fact a member of the lily family.

Many members of this extensive family are used medicinally and some are toxic, but asparagus is one that can be eaten with most beneficial effects. Raw shoots eaten before a meal are still thought to be

a reliable cure for water retention and should the shoots be out of season then tinned ones possess similar properties, although they are less powerful.

The fern-like leaf can be used dried to prepare a tea when fresh plants are unavailable. Steep 100g of asparagus leaves in 1 litre of boiling water for 10 minutes, then drink 1 cupful before meals once a day. It has a bitter flavour but can be sweetened with honey.

Basil
(Ocimum basilicum)
Family: LABIATAE

USA: sweet basil

Few culinary herbs are more hedged about by myths and legends than basil. These range from an association with a Russian youth called Vasili renowned for his beauty, to a royal connection with the Greeks and a more fanciful and slightly alarming fourteenth-century myth which would have us believe that a sprig of basil placed beneath a stone would turn into a scorpion within two or three days.

In many early writings, such as those of the sixteenth-century traveller Thomas Lupton, you will find a thousand such stories. An Italian with a scorpion breeding in his brain because he was addicted to smelling basil is one of those tales which no doubt grew substantially in the telling across the

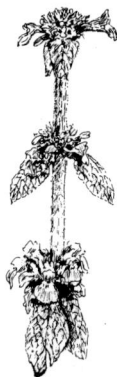

years, even before Lupton heard it. It is interesting to speculate as to the original happening . that sparked off such an unlikely story.

Basil possesses a scent and flavour enjoyed by the people of almost every continent. In India the closely related holy basil (*Ocimum sanctum*) is revered, for it is thought to hold several good spirits, and is sacred to Krishna Vishnu.

Basil is difficult to grow in British gardens; being a sub-tropical plant it abhors cold, damp winters. It is also subject to another problem which makes it difficult for herb gardeners who do not use artificial pesticides or slug and snail deterrents. Basil seems to be as attractive to these molluscs as it is to humans, and in a few evenings they will strip every leaf from a growing plant.

Breeders of *escargots* would do well to feed their charges a few leaves of basil, adding that little extra flavour to the finished dish.

Medicinally, basil has been used since Greek and Roman times as a tranquillizer and a constituent in medicaments to calm the digestion. The Japanese employed basil tea as a treatment for the common cold, and in sixteenth-century Europe an infusion of basil made by steeping 5g of the fresh plant, particularly the flowering tips, in a cupful of water was said to drive out the stuffiness caused by inflamed mucous membranes. In fact, all across the world there are remedies for fever and headaches and colds associated with this aromatic plant.

There are any number of remedies for the digestion containing basil but this one from France seems less fanciful than most. Take a clear-glass container with a tightly fitting screw top – a honey or peanut butter jar would be ideal. Fill it with roughly chopped basil leaves and flowering tips. Then pour in olive oil until it reaches the top. Allow to stand in bright sunlight for three weeks. Strain off the oil, pressing the last of it from the plant, then add this liquid to a further jar of basil. At the end of six weeks the oil will have absorbed much of the basil's fragrance and properties. A teaspoon of this oil is helpful in calming the stomach after a meal, and for constipation. There are few medicines better for restoring the tone of the intestines.

Remedies for catarrh recommend that basil leaves be crushed to a pulp and the juice expressed and snuffed up the nose. However, this could well be a hangover from the days when it was thought that spitting or copious nasal secretions carried away ill humours from the body and many leaves were used in this way to stimulate saliva or mucus.

Basil appears to be one of those aromatic plants similar to feverfew that have beneficial effects on migraine headaches. Some sufferers can be greatly helped by chewing the leaves daily to tranquillize the nervous system and prevent the tension that produces the headache in the first place.

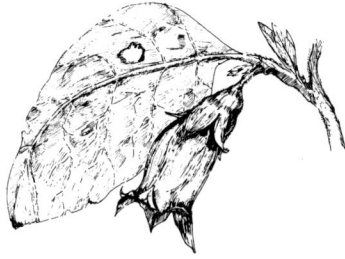

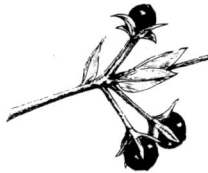

Belladonna/ Deadly nightshade

(Atropa belladonna)
Family: SOLANACEAE

Belladonna is also commonly known as deadly nightshade – and with good reason, for history is sprinkled with murders brought about with the aid of leaves and roots from this member of the potato family. Its history is long and it's likely that this was one of the first poisons used by man against his fellows.

Its common names are many and varied, but one of the most interesting is 'dwale'. This is an Anglo-Saxon word and stems from the time when it was used as a narcotic to produce a dream-like state. However, the effect was so variable as to have claimed the lives of many users. It could be said that the 'dwale time' or dream-state became permanent for them.

It is easy to confuse the various members of the nightshade family. Woody nightshade (see page 181) is quite different, and far less toxic.

The generic name, *Atropa*, derives from Atropos, one of the three fates of Greek mythology who cut man's thread of life, and the old name of 'devil's cherries' also carries a sinister significance. The name belladonna, meaning 'beautiful lady' came about because the juice was once used by Italian ladies to dilate the pupils of their eyes, giving them a doe-eyed look and supposedly rendering them more attractive. Overuse of the juice of belladonna, which contains the powerful alkaloid hyoscyamine, caused glaucoma and blindness, the retina of the eye being exposed to too much light with resulting severe impairment to sight.

The modern benefits derived from this plant are considerable, for atropine and hyoscyamine derivatives are both administered to dilate pupils in patients undergoing eye surgery and can also be used as a suppressant of salivary and biliary secretions.

This plant should never be used by anyone unqualified. It is unforgiving in action.

During medieval times when witchcraft was practised, belladonna was pressed into service to produce a series of effects attributed to possession by the devil. Symptoms were extreme talkativeness and excitability followed by loss of coordination and speech. Eventually the victim became unable to resist suggestion and would do exactly as he or she was told. A state of hysteria was next followed by convulsions, with the victim falling into a deep sleep often ending in death. Looking into the records of many sixteenth-century so-called witch trials, one detects hints of deadly nightshade poisoning in more than a few of the reported happenings. Despite the fact that belladonna is fairly common in south-east England, very few cases of poisoning occur, even though the berries are shiny black and inviting to look at.

In spite of the ferocity of the poisonous alkaloid contained in belladonna, it has served man as a constituent of medicines for many generations and was applied externally until well into the 1940s as a poultice to relieve congestion in the breasts of women who were weaning their babies.

Reference to Culpeper shows that he greatly valued belladonna for the vast range of foul ulcers his patients seemed to suffer.

Medicine derived from belladonna was popular in the United States in the 1890s as a treatment for convulsions and as a sedative for whooping cough.

Betony
(Stachys officinalis)
Family: LABIATAE

USA: betony, woundwort

Also known as wood betony, this plant, resembling a small rather aromatic stinging nettle, has been a medicinal herb for centuries from Greek and Roman times. The Greek physician Dioscorides held it in such high regard that he prescribed it for many illnesses, and Galen is quoted as saying that it cured many otherwise incurable ills.

The Romans used it extensively, and as well as being a remedy for ills caused by germs, viruses and injury, betony was also thought to be helpful before a substantial intake of alcohol to reduce the effects of drunkenness. There is no evidence that this is so, but there is

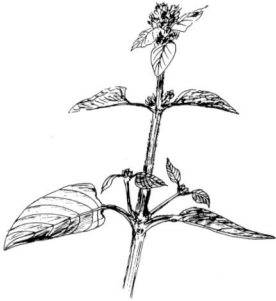

good reason to believe that betony does have certain other virtues for healing.

It has power as a diuretic and for treating headaches, particularly migraine, and has been prescribed in the past as a specific for gout and rheumatism.

In the Middle Ages it was known as 'bishop's weed', and this name is still used in some country districts. It was a regular addition to monastic herb gardens, not only for its medicinal virtues but for its usefulness as a yellow wool dye. The Saxons, too, who had strong religious connections with the soil and worshipped the earth mother, treasured betony.

Birthwort

(Aristolochia clematitis)
Family: ARISTOLOCHIACEAE

Birthwort flowers are rather strange and strong-smelling and rarely occur in the United Kingdom, although members of this family grow over much of Europe and the American continent.

The Greeks recommended this plant in an infusion for easing childbirth, and although the Doctrine of Signatures (as explained on page 13) only came to prominence in the sixteenth and seventeenth centuries, certain plants bore such a strong resemblance to parts of the human anatomy that they were automatically employed to treat problems associated with those parts.

Birthwort certainly has a superficial resemblance to the female reproductive system; the yellow flowers have long, tubular, fused petals terminating in a womb-like structure. However, it was not the flowers which were used to ease childbirth and help to bring away the placenta after delivery, but the hard tubular root, dried and ground to a powder and added to wine.

There seems to be little connection between birthwort's employment as a midwife's aid and its later

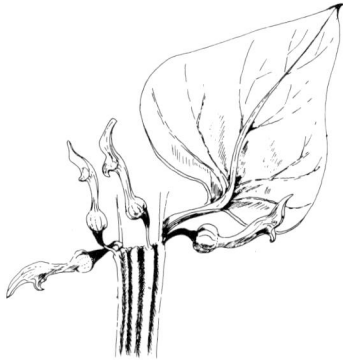

use for treating snakebite and scorpion stings, but that is how it features in many later herbals.

Other members of this family are used in America for snakebite, and the Virginian snakeroot (*Aristolochia serpentaria*) was thought to be very effective against rattlesnake bites. There are no reliable records as to the effectiveness of this treatment, but there is an interesting parallel here in that ancient Egyptian snake handlers administered an extract of a species of birthwort to calm their snakes so they could be handled without too much hazard. They too recommended birthwort as a specific against snakebite.

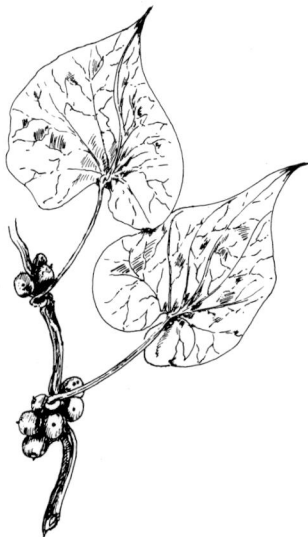

Black bryony
(Tamus communis)
Family: DIOSCOREACEAE

A member of the yam family, black bryony should not be confused with white bryony, as the two plants are completely unrelated. However, they both exhibit extremely toxic properties.

Black bryony berries are actually red and luscious when ripe, and greatly relished by birds who seem to suffer no ill effects from eating them. They are severe in their action as far as humans are concerned, however, and symptoms of black bryony poisoning include paralysis and depression of the central nervous system, which can in turn lead to death by asphyxiation.

Luckily, very few cases of death by black bryony poisoning have been recorded, for the action of the berries causes vomiting.

An extract of this plant is used homoeopathically for rheumatic pains, and the root, a far less impressive organ than the root of white bryony, is also employed for this purpose, applied as a compress to the affected joint.

Caution should be exercised here, as frequently there can be adverse skin reactions to the juice, which can cause blistering and very severe irritation. The juice can be used as an emergency styptic to stop bleeding from a wound, but care must be taken with it and as a general rule this plant should be classed with white bryony as being too dangerous for amateurs.

Black horehound

(Ballota nigra)
Family: LABIATAE

Also known as 'stinking Roger', this plant was employed in the Middle Ages for a host of medicinal purposes. Followers of the Doctrine of Signatures may have linked the unpleasant smell of this member of the nettle family with an ability to cure some less-than-pleasant sores and ulcers that were the secondary symptoms of venereal disease.

A common plant – keen gardeners would call it a weed – for the low, scrambling, rather hairy foliage is often found on disturbed land and frequently grows by the field's edge and at the side of paths. The woody hairy stems can be as much as 1m tall, although usually they grow to only half this height.

The flowers, borne at the leaf axils, are pink and typically labiate in shape with a hood. They bloom from June onwards, and the strong smell is very apparent when the plant is gathered. It's easy to see how it came to be called stinking Roger.

Medicinally horehound has a long history. Greeks and Romans used it to treat people bitten by mad dogs and for relieving spasms and nervous twitches. The method of treatment for bites was described by Dioscorides, who states that the plant should be beaten to a pulp with salt and then applied directly to the bite. It was obviously considered an effective treatment, for this remedy was used until the beginning of the twentieth century in Europe. Salt would certainly have helped to disinfect the immediate area of a wound, and the astringent action coupled with antiseptic properties may well have proved valuable in reducing infection from non-rabid animal bites.

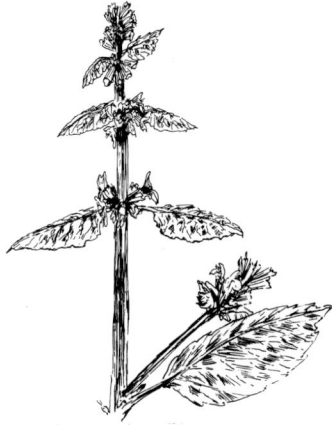

Throughout the Middle Ages and well into the seventeenth century, black horehound juice was used to relieve what we would describe today as antenatal depression and premenstrual tension. Culpeper considered it suitable for strengthening weak stomachs and correcting menstrual disorders, but it has a rather bitter astringent taste.

Many herbalists used the juice as a constituent in cough medicines and as a specific for shortness of breath. Its bitter principles were also administered to expel intestinal parasites; however, there are better worm treatments in the herbal armoury and the main value of black horehound to modern herbalists would appear to be in treating persistent coughs and nausea, because of its anti-spasmodic properties.

Blackberry
(Rubus fruticosus)
Family: ROSACEAE

Blackberry bushes have had a greater effect on the general shaping of our English landscape than almost any other plant. The sharp prickly bines are deterrent to all but the thickest hides, and few creatures, including man, will attempt to venture into a bramble thicket. In consequence blackberry has become a colonizer of open land, forming a barrier behind which tender trees and shrubs can grow and small mammals thrive safe from birds of prey and owls. In summer, when the blackberry flowers are out, a multitude of insects throngs the white-and-pink flowers, from honey and bumble bees to beautiful white admiral butterflies. Woodland economy would be quite different if blackberries were to disappear.

The fruit, so luscious and so beloved of wine and jam makers, has rich medicinal properties and is full of vitamin C and minerals, as are the leaves. The growing tips have a sharp, slightly astringent taste not unlike the unripe fruit; this is because of the presence of considerable amounts of tannin, and the tonic effect of these is appreciated by wild rabbits and by domesticated species too.

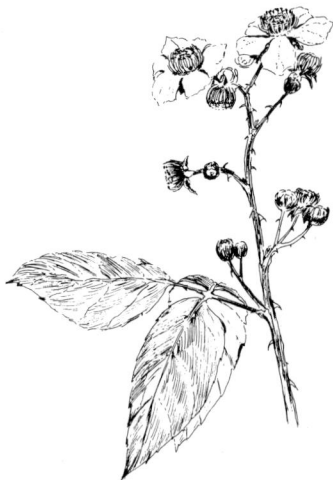

The therapeutic effects naturally occurring in blackberry shoots are excellent for digestive ailments and skin problems. The shoots are rather too astringent for human palates, but if soft growing tips are prepared by steaming and then mixed with other green vegetables they are less bitter and their tonic properties are still available.

Blackberry leaves are recommended as a general tonic and as a remedy for mild anaemia and debility. The high mineral content of the leaf is extracted by steeping 2 cupfuls of pounded fresh leaf in 1 litre of boiling water. Allow to cool, then strain and drink 2 cups a day sweetened with honey.

A similar brew is recommended as a skin lotion and as relief for some types of eczema. If this remedy is contemplated for eczema a skin test should be carried out, for eczema can have as its basis an allergic reaction to a specific allergen. Any skin test should be made on the inside of the forearm, and if there is no reaction or reddening it can be reasonably assumed that there will be no adverse effects to the lotion. It is common, in eczema, that sufferers also have a lessening of the skin's immune system, therefore total cleanliness is essential, and, of course, the blackberry lotion should be used freshly made.

Blackberries are the most commonly used natural fruit in Great Britain. Not only do they provide beneficial vitamins and minerals, they are also an excellent source of fibre. The seeds, which nature has designed to be resistant to digestive processes, are planted all over the countryside by hundreds of birds and small mammals.

The medicinal properties of the wild blackberry are also vested in domesticated varieties and in hybrids like the loganberry.

Borage
(Borago officinalis)
Family: BORAGINACEAE

Also known as 'bee bread', 'cool tankard' and, because of the shape and texture of the bristly leaves, 'ox tongue'. This plant has a long history in herbal terms. It was originally thought to have been imported to the British Isles as a medicinal herb by the Romans, but this theory is now in some doubt, as there is good reason to believe that it is a native of this country.

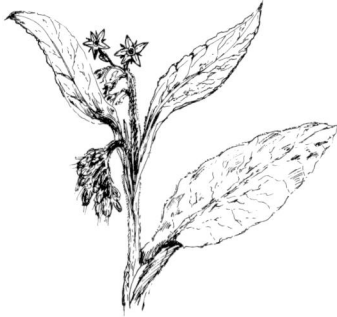

It has been cultivated for centuries and was used as an infusion to promote courage on the jousting field, a property highly valued since Greek times. It was also believed to inspire those who were about to go into battle. There are references in ancient writings to the fact that it made a man merry.

The flowers are really the only part of the plant used today, for example, for decorating wine cups. The brilliant blue petals floating on top are a highly attractive addition to any drink. The use of borage as an additive to wine and ale led to the name 'cool tankard'.

The active ingredients are mucilage, tannin and small amounts of volatile oil. The mucilage content explains why it was prescribed (mixed with fumitory) as a borage plaster for skin irritations caused by infections such as ringworm.

When taken internally it is mildly diuretic, but the power of its action is doubtful. However, the young leaves are rich in minerals, particularly calcium and potassium, and are a valuable dietary supplement when used in a salad. Only young leaves should be employed for this purpose as the older ones take on an unacceptable bristly texture.

The virtues of borage for treating eye inflammations and as a supplement to increase the flow of milk in nursing mothers have been largely discredited by modern research. Even so, it is a useful addition to a herb or wild garden, if only for its lovely flowers which are very attractive to bees.

Broom
(Cytisus scoparius)
Family: LEGUMINOSAE

The whole of the leguminous plant family seems to have been employed by man since very early times, and the power of this extensive botanical group to fix free nitrogen in the soil for the benefit of other plants has made it popular with farmers over the centuries.

Broom is one of those plants that takes over when land is left to return to nature, and on exposed soil broom bushes often play the role of protector, enriching the soil

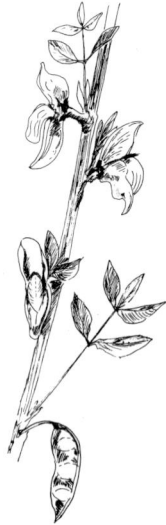

until they are shaded out as the embryo forest for which they initially provided food and shelter grows and blots out the sun.

It is an extremely useful plant, for as well as its ability to increase the soil's fertility it has various medicinal properties, the best-known being a gentle diuretic obtained from the fresh growing tips and employed in treating jaundice and dropsy. It should not be used, however, in cases of high blood pressure, as it has hypertensive effects.

It was prescribed in the past as a remedy for symptoms of rabies, though there is little evidence to back these claims in any herbals from earliest times right up to those of quite recent origin.

However, evidence does show

that a lotion made by infusing a handful of leaves and flowering tips in a half litre of boiling water for an hour relieves the irritation of insect bites and wasp stings, and the same brew can be employed as a worm treatment for round-worms. A tablespoon of the liquid mixed with a little honey should be taken on an empty stomach.

Bugle
(Ajuga reptans)
Family: LABIATAE

From his shop in Red Lion Street, Spitalfields, Culpeper dispensed bugle, also known as 'middle con-found' and 'sickle wort'. He stated that 'this herb belongeth to Dame Venus', yet it doesn't seem to have appeared in many seventeenth-century love potions.

Bugle was also supposed to have been good for the ills of Saturn, that is, for treating drunkards and such people, to use Culpeper's words, 'as gave themselves much to drinking and were troubled by strange fancies' – obviously a form of seventeenth-century DT's. Dried bugle plant was steeped in a little white wine, and this brew was supposed to be helpful in dissolving congealed blood, es-pecially that caused by such bruis-ing as might occur in a drunken fall.

It was also thought to be effec-tive in lessening danger from any 'thrusts inwardly', such as stab wounds. Even today, freshly crushed bugle leaves have some value as a plaster to relieve bruis-ing and help heal cuts.

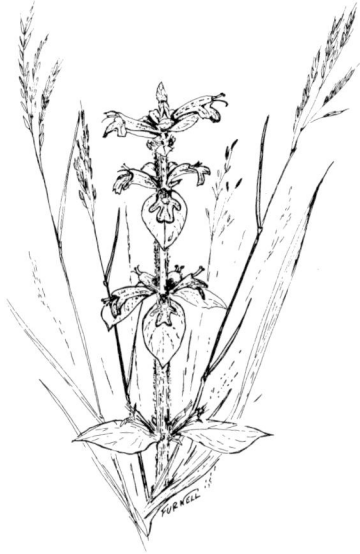

The extracted juice of the leaves is astringent and aromatic, but rather bitter. Gathered in spring, the leaves can be made into a syrup that is good for colds and sore throats, so it was a good overall cure-all.

Burdock
(Arctium lappa)
Family: COMPOSITAE

USA: beggar's buttons, clot-bur, cockle-bur, cuckoo button

Before the agricultural revolution

in the middle of the twentieth century, burdock was a common though unwelcome weed of pasture and sheep walks. It was unpopular largely because the burrs or seed heads (that part of the plant from which it takes its name) caused loss of value to fleeces. Sheep wandered into patches of burdock to graze and the burrs stuck firmly to the wool, tangling it and creating problems in preparation of the fleece for spinning.

Farmers and shepherds waged a constant war against this tough plant, yet it thrived. Only since the advent of selective weed killers has burdock retreated, until now it's no longer common over much of its former range. Burdock now most often occurs in suburban gardens and parks.

Despite the dislike of farmers, burdock has been treasured by herbalists for generations as one of the most valuable herbs of the field.

The root of this handsome plant can grow to a substantial size, up to 1m long in good soil, and as thick as a man's wrist. It can be eaten as a vegetable, boiled and served in much the same way as parsnip or salsify, but it has little to recommend it from a gastronomic point of view although it is rich in vitamins and minerals.

The stems of young plants can be candied, or skinned and boiled in the same manner as asparagus, and when so prepared are sweet-tasting and nourishing. The young leaves can be steamed and served with a cheese sauce and the tenderest leaves chopped and added to a salad. These methods of preparing burdock retain valuable amounts of vitamins A, B and C, as well as iron and calcium.

Seeds are extracted from the burrs by drying naturally until they fall when the burrs are turned upside down. Kept for sprouting, they are a novel addition to winter salads.

Burdock was and indeed still is used by herbalists to treat skin irritations, and in the past it was a remedy for the effects of tertiary syphilis. King Henry III was said to have benefited from treatment with burdock.

Skin problems such as ringworm and sores may respond to a lotion of burdock root prepared as follows. Put 60g of thoroughly cleaned and sliced root into $\frac{1}{2}$ litre of boiling water. Allow to cool and then discard the root. If it is to be taken internally, 1 tablespoon should be mixed with 1 tablespoon of honey and added to a small cup of milk 3 times a day after meals. Externally, spread 1 tablespoonful on a cloth and bind over the affected part for several hours. This should reduce external irritation.

However, many skin eruptions may be allergic reactions, so it's best to carry out a skin test first. The inside of the forearm is a good test area and if there is any irritation or redness within an hour of application then don't use. If you get a skin reaction it would also be

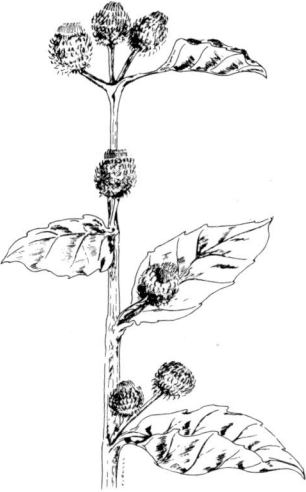

be more distressing than loss of hair.

However, one which comes from France and is widely used on the Continent, is to rub in equal quantities of pounded burdock root, fresh burdock leaves and wine vinegar. This is said to be stimulating and will help keep the scalp healthy.

Lastly, the peeled stem and root can be liquidized together with a quantity of young leaves to produce a vitamin-rich health drink. If taken regularly it can lower blood-sugar levels by reducing the amount of insulin secreted, so sweeten with a little honey to counterbalance this effect.

unwise to take this preparation internally.

Gypsy herbalists regard burdock as a specific for rheumatism, particularly in the form of a poultice of fresh leaves that have been steamed and allowed to cool to blood heat and then applied to the affected joints for about two hours. The causes of joint pains are complex and wide-ranging, however, so there is no guarantee that this will have the desired effect on all types of rheumatic pain.

The same applies to burdock leaves prepared as a scalp lotion to prevent your hair falling out, although some people swear by it. If you want to try it, soak 20g of fresh leaves in 1 litre of hot water and massage into the scalp night and morning. But beware, as there are a number of remedies for toning the scalp, some of which would

Cabbage

(Brassica oleracea)
Family : CRUCIFERAE

In some parts of Devon and Cornwall wild brassica, or cabbage, grows on sea cliffs and southerly banks. Cabbage has been cultivated by man since prehistoric times, though whether as a food or as a medicinal herb is debatable. Today cabbage is recognized as a valuable source of minerals, and providing that it is steamed lightly and not boiled with bicarbonate of soda, as was popular in grandmother's time, it is one of the best natural sources of vitamin C.

It's difficult to think of cabbage in any other way than as one of the vegetables in 'meat and two veg',

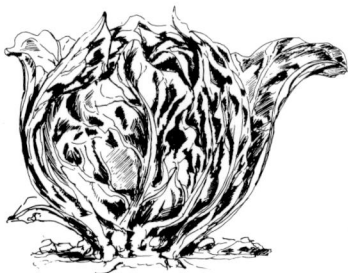

but in the past it was known variously as 'doctor of the poor' and 'gift from heaven'.

The leaves were applied to varicose ulcers, wounds and even gangrene. Savoy cabbage was most favoured for this. Choose leaves as green as possible, wash them thoroughly, then remove the middle rib and crush the smaller ribs by hammering them with a wooden mallet. Warm the leaves and apply several layers to any area requiring treatment. Hold in place with a bandage and change the application every four hours.

Coughs and hoarseness were treated with cabbage syrup prepared in the following way. Take a red cabbage and liquidize either in a blender or foodmill, or by pounding and pressing to extract the juice. This juice should be strained and weighed and half its weight in honey added to it. Simmer the mixture of cabbage juice and honey over a low heat until it reaches the consistency of syrup. Several doses of 2 teaspoonfuls can be taken in quick succession with no harmful effects, and it is not unpleasant in taste.

To heal blisters, boil cabbage leaves in milk and apply when cool. You can also continue to boil the milk and cabbage together until the leaves reach a jelly-like consistency; applied as a hot poultice, this was said to relieve lumbago and muscular pain.

These are only a few of the many remedies for which cabbage earned its name of 'doctor plant'.

Caraway
(Carum carvi)
Family: UMBELLIFERAE

Confectionery, rather than herbalism, comes to mind when we think of caraway, as the seeds are used to flavour sweets and cakes. Indeed, ancient Egyptians flavoured their sweetmeats with it, and in the time of Elizabeth I of England the seeds were candied with sugar and honey and eaten with baked apples.

Most cookery books mention caraway and it certainly adds a characteristic flavour to any recipe.

However, it was also known as a medicinal plant for relieving stomach disorders and as a mild stimulant for promoting good digestion.

The Pharmaceutical Pocket Book, published by the direction of the Council of the Pharmaceutical Society of Great Britain, lists a tincture of aromatic cardamom, the extracted oil of caraway, as a medicine for upset stomachs.

It is one of a large and valued

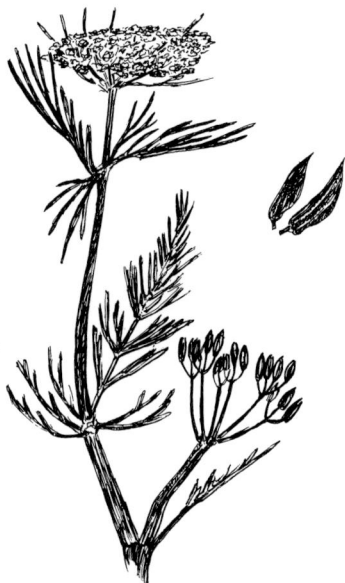

Under certain circumstances wild caraway leaves could be confused with that other Roman favourite, the poisonous hemlock, and *if you are at all doubtful leave well alone*; a mistake could easily prove fatal.

In the wild, caraway is rare, but although it is at the very northern limit of its climatic tolerance range it can be found growing wild in England. It is easy to grow in a kitchen garden or in a border and is an attractive, stately plant with feathery leaves and white umbels of flowers. It should be sown in early spring in a greenhouse or in a propagator and pricked out into individual pots for planting when frosts are less likely.

family to which many well-known culinary favourites belong. This includes such plants as celery, carrot, fennel – another aromatic herb – and also parsley.

Caraway resembles common cow parsley, which grows profusely in early spring hedgerows, and like carrot, it has a fleshy root where it stores food for the winter. This root can be ground and mixed with pastry to make a type of cake which is extremely nourishing and rich in minerals. In Norway and Sweden today there are still recipes for caraway bread which are thought to owe their origins to the Romans, and caraway leaves are still put into sandwiches to add a little savour in much the same way as parsley is used to flavour sauces.

Carline thistle
(Carlina vulgaris)
Family: COMPOSITAE

Certain plants in the herbal armoury have a long, long history and such a one is carline thistle. It is a native of impoverished chalk downland; where the herbage is low carline thrives.

It is an odd plant in that the flowering head appears to be dead when it is actually in full flower. A glossy fawn and gold, the sharply spined flower has a faintly metallic sheen which adds to its rather unreal appearance. When a carline thistle is in full bloom the stem is short, often only about 7–8cm tall. The flower heads can be dried and

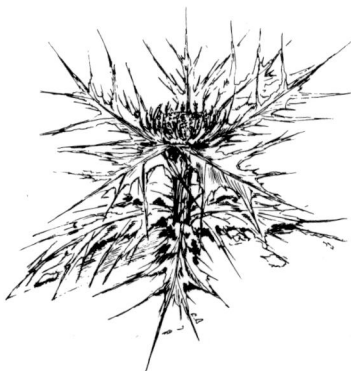

used in flower arrangements, but they are becoming rare now, as their natural habitat of chalk downland is vanishing.

It is thought that the name 'carline' is associated with the famous king of the Franks and later Holy Roman Emperor, Charlemagne. The French herbalist Jean Ruel wrote in his *De Historia Stirpium* in 1536 that whilst the Emperor and his troops were under siege in a castle the troops were stricken with plague and an angel revealed the thistle to him as a remedy.

There is little documentary evidence to prove that carline thistle would be of value in cases of bubonic plague, but it still has a great following in southern France where peasants gather young flowers and eat them in much the same way as artichokes.

The leaves were formerly used to curdle milk, but it is the stubby thick brown root that is most prized by herbalists. This is gathered and dried before being broken into pieces and adminis-

tered as a calming agent for stomach ailments.

To prepare an infusion, steep 30g of root in 1 litre of boiling water for 10 minutes, then bring back to the boil for a further 10 minutes. Allow to cool and strain. A wineglass of this brew should be taken before meals.

For skin irritation and eczema, steep 30g of root in $\frac{1}{2}$ litre of cheap white wine for a period of 10 days. A small wineglass to be taken before the midday meal.

Carrot
(Daucus carota)
Family: UMBELLIFERAE

(Pictured: wild carrot)

Carrots are humble vegetables and have long been associated with health farms. Whenever one reads a satirical exposition on treating obesity or 'getting fit', there is nearly always a reference to carrot juice as part of a regime of exercises and diet.

During the Second World War, carrots were considered excellent for promoting good night vision and care of the eyes in general. In fact there is some basis for believing that carrots, which are rich in mineral salts and vitamins as well as the yellow/orange compound carotene, are good for general health and well-being, and eyes are great indicators of health and fitness.

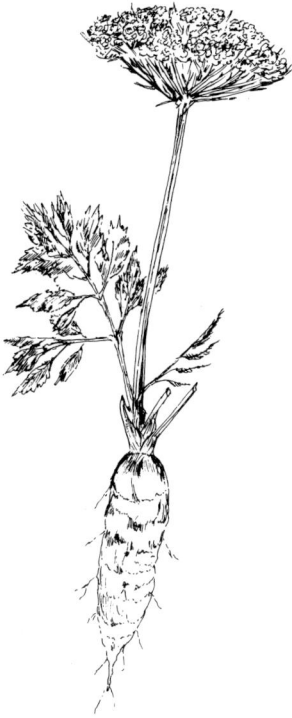

fertilizer and without toxins, carrots are beneficial above all other vegetables.

Carrot juice is reputed to be of great value to anyone suffering from anaemia, and in some clinics carrot juice has been recommended as a supplement in treating cancer and other drastically debilitating diseases.

Grated carrot root is very good for making poultices to relieve burns and reduce the pain caused by boils and whitlows. Raw grated carrot used to be employed in conjunction with worming agents to render them more efficient and to remedy some of their toxic effects.

Carrots are considered to be beneficial to the liver, and red blood corpuscles have been shown to increase as a result of a diet rich in raw carrot. In the past it was employed to treat jaundice, and ulcers of the digestive tract. The juice is also strongly recommended for kidney troubles and urine retention.

A word of warning here. If you intend to use much raw carrot in your diet it is best to grow them yourself, if you have sufficient ground, or to buy organically grown carrots where toxic chemicals have been shunned. Modern bulk-producers of carrots use chemical pesticides in order to ensure heavy cropping and freedom from attack by carrot root fly. These chemicals are likely to accumulate in body tissues, to your detriment.

However, grown with natural

Grated root applied to the eyelids in cases of severe styes is quite effective, and a poultice made from pulped raw carrot root with the addition of some finely chopped or pulverized carrot leaf is said to provide a better beauty dressing for tired skin than anything that comes out of a tube. Apply the carrot pulp as a face pack daily for a week. The results are often very satisfactory. However, before using any plant-based face packs please first test for allergic reaction by applying a small amount of the pack to an area of skin on the inside of the forearm. If any reddening develops, do not use.

Catmint

(Nepeta cataria x faassenii)
Family: LABIATAE

USA: catnip

As its name suggests, catmint, often referred to in ancient herbals as nepeta and by Gerard as nep, is associated with cats, who are said to find the smell irresistible.

It contains metatabilacetone, a chemical that does appear to have a tranquillizing effect on members of the cat family, and this same compound seems to have a similar effect on humans. This may be why it has found favour as a natural tranquillizer since Roman times. There is a story of an executioner in France who could not carry out his gruesome task until he had calmed his nerves by chewing catmint root.

It is a wild plant from the dry regions of southern France and is considered originally to have been a hybrid which has now become naturalized throughout much of Europe and the Mediterranean area. Legend has it that catmint was brought to these islands by the Romans, who introduced many herbs during their occupation, but there is a distinct possibility that it

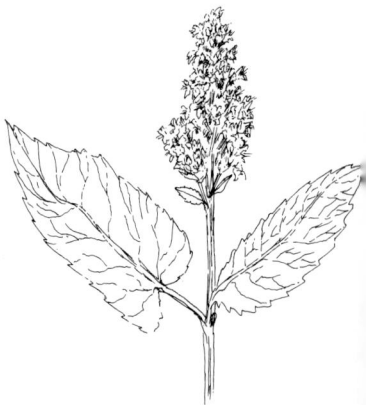

was part of our flora before that time.

It grows wild in many parts of southern England where chalk soil predominates and is smaller, more delicate and less rampant in its growth than the majority of other labiates. The finely toothed leaves and pretty blue flowers which open in July and August have made this mint more favoured as a bedding plant than as a herb.

In the thirteenth century it was used to flavour meat, for it imparts a delicate pungency to food, and monastery gardens were well supplied with nep, which was encouraged as much for its value to bees as for any other virtue.

Medicinally, it was prescribed to relieve colic in young children and as an ingredient in cough remedies and for colds and giddy headaches. However, the main virtues of catmint seem to be calming and cooling, and lowering temperature by promoting perspiration; hence its frequent presence in remedies for coughs and colds.

A strong tea made from dried leaves – a handful to $\frac{1}{2}$ litre of boiling water infused for 10 minutes and sweetened with a little honey – is recommended for stomach cramps and to promote a feeling of general well-being.

And cats both large and small are soothed by the chemical compound contained in this plant; it is sometimes used to quieten big cats in zoological gardens

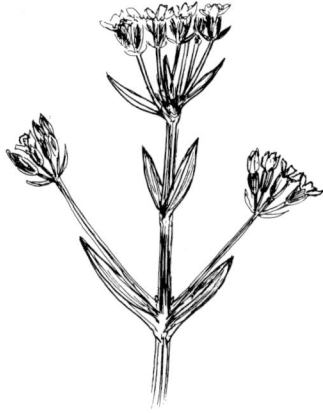

Centaury

(Centaurium erythraea)
Family: GENTIANACEAE

'The universal purifier' was the grandiose title given to centaury, a small, rather attractive, many-flowered plant. It was also called 'century', and 'feverwort'.

In the sixteenth and seventeenth centuries it was thought to be a specific for many contagious diseases and, to quote from an old herbal, 'it causes the bile to flow, cures jaundice, strengthens the liver and the stomach'. It is clear they believed it would cure most ills.

The truth is slightly less dramatic, however, even though the bitter principles extracted from the flower heads are known to have a mildly stimulating effect on the digestive system, increasing the flow of both digestive juices and saliva.

It would appear from ancient herbals that our ancestors' digestive systems must have been under considerable pressure. Most of the old books and treatises on medicine deal in great depth with remedies to ease stomach ache, and since everyone, from the highest in the land to the meanest peasant, suffered from intestinal parasites, preoccupation with affairs of the digestive system must have assumed an importance second only to affairs of the heart.

Centaury had no romantic connotations, but it was certainly recommended for killing tapeworms. Its greatest benefit appears to have been that, unlike many other potions popular at the time, even if it didn't do much good, it was relatively harmless.

Centaury got its name from Ancient Greece. According to legend, the centaur Chiron, who taught surgery to the god of medicine,

Aesculapius, used the herb to heal a wound inflicted on him by the god Hercules, who had accidentally shot him in the foot with a poisoned arrow. From that time forward the herb was revered by many cultures, from the Romans, who believed it had magic powers to drive away snakes, to the Gauls who, in the Dark Ages, used it as a snakebite antidote. The results obtained are not recorded!

Stripping away myth from reality is always difficult, but it is a fact that centaury makes a good skin lotion. Infuse 1 tablespoon of dried flowers in $\frac{1}{2}$ litre of boiling water, stand until cool, then strain. This same lotion when diluted half-and-half in freshly boiled and cooled water is said to tone up the digestive system.

Chamomile
(Matricaria chamomilla, Matricaria recutita)
Family: COMPOSITAE

USA: bowman, chamomile

Chamomile is one of the most popular herb teas. It seems to soothe the soul and lighten the spirit.

Herbal teas used to be very popular prior to the introduction of imported tea from India and Ceylon (now Sri Lanka) and chamomile tea is still a favourite among herbal teas, especially in Europe.

This rather insignificant-looking member of the daisy family

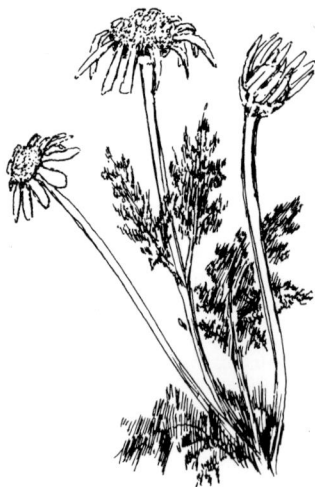

used to be found all over the southern half of England and is thought to have been introduced to the USA by German immigrants. You can still find it growing where cereals are not predominant, but it is a tender weed unable to stand the potent chemicals we spray on our land. Its near relative, scentless mayweed (*Matricaria maritima*), looks very similar but does not have the power of its sweetly scented cousin, although in some country districts chamomile used to be known as scented mayweed.

Medicinally, chamomile is employed to relieve kidney and liver disorders and painful periods. Both the Greeks and the Romans considered it the best herb for menstrual disorders, and the flowers are the part used, although the level of active ingredient is rather weak. In order to make a brew of sufficient strength, steep 1 tablespoonful of dried flowers in a cup of boiling water, cover with a saucer, and allow to brew in a warm place for 10 minutes; strain and drink. It is still considered excellent for soothing the cramps of painful periods.

There are many references from all over the Mediterranean countries to the use of chamomile flowers in olive oil for muscle cramps. This oil can be prepared by filling a glass jar with flowers and adding enough olive oil to take up any space in the bottle. Screw down the cap tightly and leave in the sun for 3 weeks, adding more oil and flowers as the mixture settles. Alternatively, you can heat the jar carefully in a saucepan for an hour to extract the active ingredients from the flowers. If you have time, however, it's better to leave it in the sun. Strain off the oil from the flowerheads, then press them to extract the last drop of oil. It is now ready to be rubbed on inflamed joints or strained muscles.

Chamomile has a long involvement in the annals of English history. It was one of the nine sacred herbs of the Saxons, and widely administered as a sedative and calming agent for the stomach. In later times it was valued as a strewing herb; its strong and long-lasting scent was greatly appreciated in the insanitary halls of castles and great houses. It was also burned as a form of domestic incense to keep foul smells at bay.

Today it is taken as a sedative drink or put into a tonic bath. A large sachet of chamomile flowers may be added to bath water, or alternatively a sachet of flowers is steeped in a pre-heated jug of boiling water for 15 minutes and the water is then added to the bath.

Chamomile oil in hair lotions and shampoos is extremely popular, and a final rinse prepared as for the bath lotion but cooled is said to be most superior for retaining the lustre of blond hair in a dusty city environment.

Cleavers/ Goosegrass
(Galium aparine)
Family: RUBIACEAE

USA: catchweed bedstraw

Mention goosegrass to keen vegetable gardeners, and medicinal values will be far from their minds. It is an exceptionally difficult weed to eradicate from cultivated ground without recourse to powerful chemical weedkillers.

It is closely related to that useful strewing herb, lady's bedstraw, and in common with other members of the family, can curdle milk; hence its country names of 'cheese rennet' and 'cheese rent herb'.

A strange, climbing, scrambling plant, it is capable of covering considerable areas of ground with its square stems armed with small,

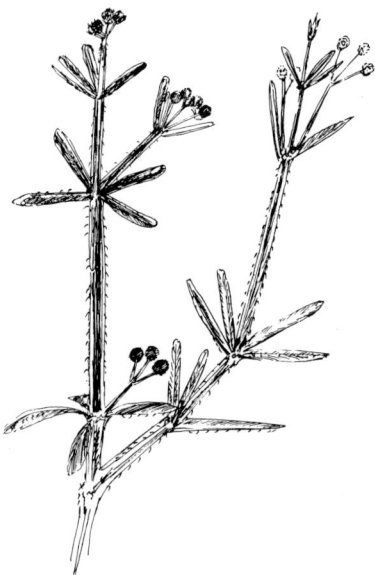

sharp hooks which catch and cling — hence the name 'cleavers', 'scratchweed' or 'sticky willy'. Sharp hooks on the seeds enable the plant to spread its seed by way of animals, as they will catch on fur and fleece to drop later at a new site ready to grow profusely.

Goosegrass stems are rich in silica and are said to be good for bones, especially after a break. Crushed and infused in boiling water, they were also formerly used as a remedy for gallstones. There is little real evidence to suggest any therapeutic effect on either the urinary or biliary system, although it is currently employed by medical herbalists to treat urinary system problems

such as cystitis. They also use it for swollen lymph glands and skin disease.

In the past both stem and root have been applied to stay bleeding from open cuts and grazes, and under difficult circumstances a temporary dressing may be made from crushed stems until a more suitable one can be obtained. The high acid content in the plant will cause smarting on a graze, but there is reason to believe that this herb is of genuine value as an emergency dressing for minor wounds, and as it's also very common, you don't have to dry it for storage but can use it fresh.

Coltsfoot
(Tussilago farfara)
Family: COMPOSITAE

In ancient times peasants looked to coltsfoot in early spring as a sovereign remedy for coughs. After all, it's not so long ago that bronchitis was called the 'English disease' because the English were the most frequent sufferers, due to climate, industrial conditions, and inadequate housing for the mass of working people.

Coltsfoot must have been greatly valued by the herbalists of old, for it has a host of country names, most of which, like 'bull's foot', 'horse hoof' and 'hall foot', refer to the appearance of the leaf, which is large, sea-green and shaped like a hoofprint in mud. One of its other

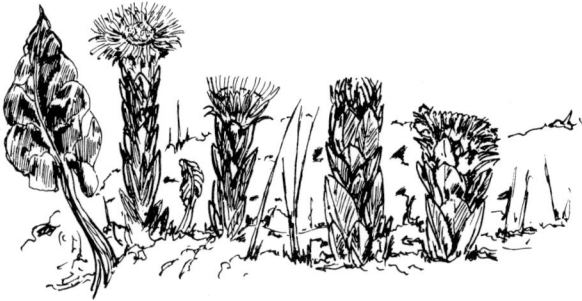

names, 'son before the father', refers to the plant's habit of flowering and setting seed before the leaves have unfurled from the rootstock.

It flowers very early in the year; even February's winter sun will bring some of the scaly stems up towards the light. The brilliant yellow flowers resemble dandelions, as does the down which carries the seeds away from the parent plant with the first springtime wind, and the plant is able to colonize large areas of land by this strategy.

The rootstock is thick and spreading and was used to prepare a medicine for heart ailments, although there is little evidence of its effectiveness. Cardiac conditions are in any case too potentially dangerous to attempt to treat yourself.

It was as a cough remedy that the plant was best known, and the Greeks and later the Romans drank infusions of the flowers and stems for persistent coughs. They believed that the flowering spikes had special curative powers because they bloomed so early in the year, at a time when coughs were at their worst. However, it appears that the same expectorant properties for coughs and chest infections are present in the large leaves. There is some evidence, too, that the plant contains an antispasmodic, the effective constituents of which are faradial and phytosterol, and would therefore be of value in treating chest infections.

To prepare a tea for cough and cold symptoms add 1–3 tablespoons of dried coltsfoot leaves and flowers to 1 litre of cold water, bring to the boil for 5 minutes, then allow to cool. A little honey will improve the taste, which can be rather bitter.

An infusion of leaves and flowers is recommended for wounds that are slow to heal. The leaves can also be bruised and placed over a cut as an emergency plaster.

Comfrey
(Symphytum officinale)
Family: BORAGINACEAE

USA: common comfrey, knitbone

Comfrey is a very popular herbal remedy, known variously as 'cure-all', 'knitbone', 'bone-set' and 'bruise wort'. With all these names there is little wonder that its prime use is to promote healing of fractures. It has been employed in this way for over two thousand years.

The name 'comfrey' appears to date from Roman times. Pliny described it as a plant of healing that grew in water or by water and caused wounds to grow together; he called it *confevere*. By the fourteenth century the Latin name *conforye* had been applied to it, and this was but a short step to comfrey.

One of the tallest members of the borage family, it grows well over 1m in height and the large bristly leaves and tall stems shoot up rapidly until the flowers form in hanging clusters. The flowers vary considerably in colour, from bluish-purple through red to yellow and pure white.

Comfrey rewards the grower with a number of benefits. Some herbals and books on foods from the countryside state that comfrey leaves are edible and make a pleasant addition to salad, but the leaves would have to be picked when the plant is very young, as sharp hairs cover both leaf and stem and are irritating, not at all appetizing. In fact the hairs are there for just that purpose, as a defence mechanism, but I believe they can be cooked and that they have a flavour reminiscent of cucumber.

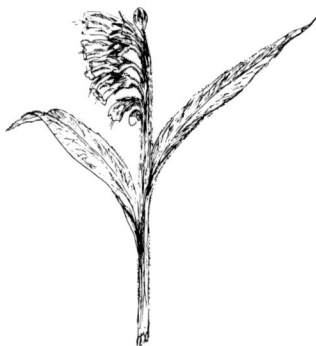

Medicinally, the leaves can be employed as a bandage to heal cuts and bring out bruises, but the root appears to contain the most healing power. As well as being rich in mucilage and tannin, it contains allantoin, particularly in the flowering tops, and a number of alkaloids that appear to be beneficial to living tissue and do seem to promote rapid healing.

The root is collected and dried and ground to a powder to be administered internally or externally for a variety of healing roles.

Comfrey has been employed to heal stomach ulcers, and for all internal uses, including bruises and broken bones, 2 tablespoons of powdered root are heated to simmering point in 1 litre of water then allowed to cool. Take 3 times a day for 3 days. It can have a purgative effect and should not be taken for long periods, or in strong concentrations.

Externally, the root is applied as a poultice. Use the same concentration and bind to the skin on a cloth as hot as is comfortable. There is little benefit in too much heat.

This treatment was popular for gout, where powdered root was drunk as a medicine and compresses were applied to an affected area. The results seem to have been satisfactory, for this remedy has stood the test of time. Comfrey for bone-healing is still used by most homoeopaths and medical herbalists, and an extract of the plant is available from some health food stores.

When fresh roots are in plentiful supply, make a paste by crushing peeled roots; it's considered an excellent salve for healing cuts and helping to reduce pain, swelling and discolouration caused by bruises. This paste is also recommended in some herbals for treating varicose veins.

Comfrey is easily grown from seed in a herb garden, although, being a large plant, when full grown it will shade out many low-growing members sharing the plot. However, it rewards you by providing a plentiful supply of green compost, for when the root is harvested both stems and leaves can be dug into the garden, especially in trenches for growing root crops. The yield is often higher than usual, as the fibre in the stems, which rots down less quickly than the leaf, helps to open heavy soils and provides substance in light soils.

Cowslip
(Primula officinalis, Primula veris)
Family: PRIMULACEAE

These low-growing plants with tall stems bearing a head of golden flowers were a common sight in the countryside before the modern agricultural revolution. Now they grow in only a few places on the downlands of southern England or along the margins of ancient woodland, and in Europe, where there is more undisturbed grassland. In parts of Dorset and Devon there are still cowslip meadows, though they are few and far between.

Cowslip has a host of country names, the best-known and most widely used being 'paigles', thought to be of Anglo-Saxon origin. Other Anglo-Saxon names are 'cuy lippe' and 'cooslip'. Some of the names have a biblical significance, like 'St Peter's keys', 'herb Peter' and 'virgin keys', probably arising because the flower heads were thought to resemble the bunch of keys carried by St Peter. There are also many non-Christian names, including 'fairies' basin', 'fairies' cup', 'drelip', 'peggle' and 'cowflop'.

Medicinally, it was held in high regard, and two other names were

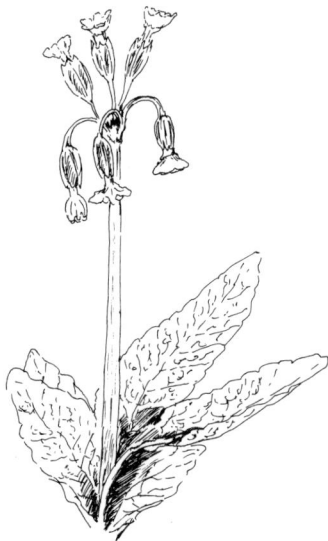

given to it: 'palseywort' and 'herba paralysis', giving some indication as to its uses.

It was prescribed as a remedy for palsy, vertigo and conditions of the middle ear leading to loss of balance, convulsions, rheumatic illnesses and liver infections. It was also applied externally as an ointment for removing freckles and softening the skin.

Even the well-known country posset, cowslip wine, wasn't taken only as an intoxicant, but as a tonic and sedative as well. The flowers are used for this brew, and there are a number of recipes, all requiring a large quantity of petals, so unless you grow them yourself it wouldn't be possible to gather enough. However, an alternative calling for fewer flowers is to candy them. Layer flowers in a jar alternately with sugar. This delicate medicament is taken a teaspoonful at a time after meals, and also makes a pleasant sweet with cream.

Flowers and leaves used to be eaten, with young leaves being cooked in much the same way as any other tender vegetable by steaming gently for a period of ten minutes to retain colour and flavour.

The root contains the highest concentration of the active principle. A mixture of dried leaf, flower and grated root (10g of each) steeped in 1 litre of water for 1 hour, then slowly brought to the boil for 3 minutes and allowed to cool before straining, was considered mildly calming for the stomach and also used in many parts of Europe for relieving bronchial spasms. Being mildly diuretic, it is often recommended for rheumatism and urinary tract disorders. The dose is 1 cupful of mixture as above 3 times a day before meals.

The sweet honey-flavoured flowers can be made into cowslip oil by putting a handful of fresh flowers and a handful of fresh, thoroughly washed chopped root into 1 litre of olive oil. Leave to stand in strong sunlight in a sealed jar for 6 weeks, then strain and store for future use on bruises and dry skin.

Cowslip is an excellent herb, but the leaves can cause an allergic reaction (primula rash) when in direct contact with sensitive skin.

It is easy to propagate from seed. Chill the seed in a tray of damp sharp sand in the fridge for about a month before sowing. Sadly, the scent from cowslip flowers, although sweet, is fleeting and vanishes on drying, as does the aniseed scent of the fresh chopped root.

Primrose
(Primula vulgaris)
Family: PRIMULACEAE

Primroses have very similar properties to cowslips and can be substituted in most remedies calling for cowslip.

In addition, they were once employed to treat intestinal parasites. 50g of whole crushed root is infused in hot water for one hour, then strained. A cupful of this 'tea' was recommended by herbalists, particularly gypsies, to be taken before breakfast.

Crab apple
(Malus sylvestris)
Apple
(Malus pumila) (pictured)
Family: ROSACEAE

How very true the old adage is, 'An apple a day keeps the doctor away.' It would be even more appropriate if the word 'dentist' were substituted for 'doctor'. Along with regular brushing,

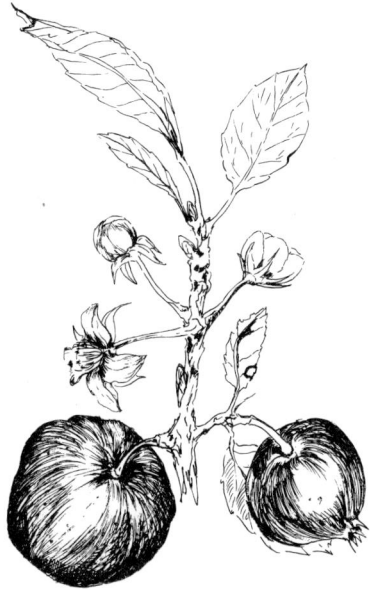

munching an apple after meals helps keep gums and teeth in good order.

Apples contain a number of minerals and vitamins, along with dietary fibre, which has just become fashionable again. They also have a good supply of fruit sugars for energy.

The Hesperides were nymphs chosen to guard the golden apples of Greek mythology, and apples feature in religions and myths from all over the world. The apple in the Garden of Eden may actually have been a fig, changed to an apple by medieval translators, and there are many nursery rhymes which feature apples as symbols of attainment.

Apples have been cultivated for many centuries, and stem originally from 'crab' or wild apple (*Malus sylvestris*), which used to be a common hedgerow plant, but has now declined as mile after mile of English country hedgerow is grubbed up. Wild crab apple bears hardy fruits, which are usually bitter, and high in tannin and malic acid, and which in the past formed a major part of autumn's wild fruit crop for peasants who turned them into preserves and alcoholic drinks. Where the trees are common, the fruits are still used for crab apple jelly.

Crab apples also form part of the staple diet of wild creatures of the countryside. Apart from providing fruit in autumn, the rough bark and leaves give shelter to insects, and crab apple trees are favoured nesting sites for small birds.

The crab apple family is distributed world-wide. The Chinese crab apple (*Malus spectabilis*) was cultivated in China from earliest times as an ornamental tree, and the hupeh crab (*Malus hupehensis*) grows right across India and Asia to the Chinese mainland and is valued for its leaves, which are gathered in spring and dried for use in red tea.

Early settlers in the United States prized the native apples of sweet crab (*Malus coronaria*) and the Oregon crab (*Malus fusca*) not so much for their fruit (though this was doubtless used) as for the very hard tight-grained heavy wood. This they carved into tools and handles: anything, in fact, that had to endure heavy wear and tear.

Apple wood is one of the best timbers for decorative furniture, but because the average branch size is small and the trunks rarely straight, it was confined to country chairs and small items of furniture for the farm or kitchen.

The grated raw flesh of sweet apples is an excellent remedy for diarrhoea and one easily taken by children, being pleasant-tasting, and there's an old remedy for bronchitis or severe coughs and sore throats dating from Tudor times and consisting of an apple baked with honey and served mashed with butter. Sounds delicious!

Fresh apple juice forms the basis of many health cures, and it's a good practice to drink a glassful everyday. It will supply many of the vitamins and minerals lacking in the average modern diet.

Apple has been used since Roman times to treat skin ailments, and the word pomade is thought to be derived from an unguent prepared from pulped apple, cloves, and lanolin (derived from sheep's wool) which Roman ladies applied to their skins to keep it clear and supple.

Finally, always choose those apples that are as nature intended them, not spotless ones covered in protecting fungicides and insecticides. Wash all apples, except those you grow yourself, to remove any impurities from the skin, and do not peel them.

Daisy
(Bellis perennis)
Family: COMPOSITAE

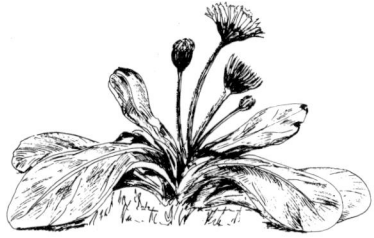

There are not many gardens where daisies fail to bloom, and, indeed, should they cease to open their flowers on lawns and playing fields, it would cause consternation among the industries which produce chemicals to control them and implements to uproot these low-growing perennials. Yet they still come up smiling, despite the endeavours of a million gardeners.

The name 'daisy' is thought to have its roots in Anglo-Saxon *daeges eage*, meaning 'day's eye', possibly because the flower closes at dusk. The name eventually became corrupted to 'daisy'.

Few plants are more able to adapt to landscape and soil type than daisy. They are high in magnesium, and perfectly edible if found on uncontaminated ground. The thick, fleshy spoon-shaped leaves may be eaten as a salad vegetable or cooked lightly to retain their mineral content and served in butter.

Medicinally, daisy has fallen from general use, although it was prescribed in ancient herbals for a host of diseases associated with the liver and spleen. Externally, it was recommended for eczema and wounds that were slow to heal, and was applied as a dressing for wounds on the battlefield. However, records show that its main purpose was for treating bruises and bloodclots, and also pleurisy and pneumonia.

The plant was crushed and steeped in a little water, then boiled for a short time to make a tea for relieving migraine, and there are references to daisy juice being snuffed up the nose to promote sneezing, which was thought to be a good way of mitigating some ailments.

One rather strange daisy remedy may have sprung from the plant's diminutive size and its preference for remaining close-growing under most soil and climatic conditions. In medieval times daisy juice in milk was fed to puppies to restrict their growth, and the same was said to have been done to children, for lap dogs and very small children were fashionable. In fact, there appears to be nothing in daisy root, leaf or flower which suggests any growth-inhibiting factor. Dogs could have been kept small through breeding and children were probably small because of poor nutrition.

Dandelion
(Taraxacum officinale)
Family: COMPOSITAE

USA: blowball, common dandelion, lion's tooth, peasant's clock

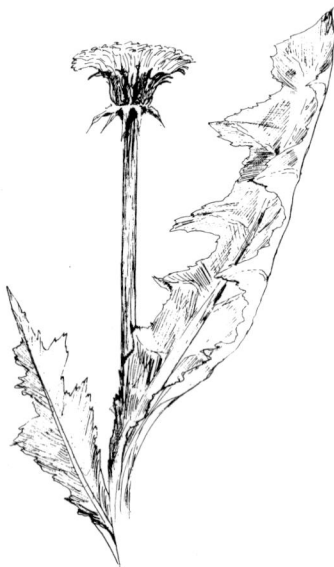

Dandelions are best known for their diuretic properties and the common name 'piss-a-bed' and the French *pissenlit* are indicative of this property. There is little doubt that the plant does promote the flow of urine to a marked degree, and it was as a treatment for dropsy, liver ailments, kidney troubles and diseases of the urinary tract that dandelions were employed for many hundreds of years.

It is one of a small group of plants that is self-fertilizing. Dandelions can produce fertile seeds without any assistance from insects or other pollinators and this has allowed them to become one of the most successful plants of both countryside and towns. Even the rush of air that accompanies motor traffic along our great arterial roads has allowed dandelions to colonize roadsides in spring through the medium of their parachute seeds.

The characteristic 'dandelion clock' seed head is incorporated in folklore all over Europe and parts of North America. In Europe, unmarried girls used to predict how many years they would have to wait before marriage by how many times they had to blow to completely clear the down from a seed head. The predictions were probably of little value to these maidens, but greatly assisted the dispersal of dandelion seeds.

The medicinal value of dandelion is still to be adequately explored. There is evidence to support the fact that this interesting plant may have properties as yet untapped, and considering how common it is, it's surprising that the edible nature of the foilage is so little exploited. Blanched under a flowerpot or upturned bucket or can, dandelions make a pleasant salad vegetable, but in early spring young unblanched leaves can be gathered and eaten, and are particularly nutritious, as they contain those minerals usually removed by blanching, especially manganese. Young spring leaves are rich in many minerals, as well as vitamins C and B, and have considerable food value.

In the past they have been used to treat gout and other conditions caused by an excess of uric acid in the body. To prepare an infusion for general liverishness and sluggish digestion a cupful of dried chopped whole plant is steeped in a litre of water overnight, then brought to the boil for five minutes. Allow to cool, strain and drink a cupful before breakfast. This will allow the diuretic properties to abate before bedtime.

The root is well known as a substitute for coffee, and larger roots are gathered to prepare this drink. Wash and split them to promote drying, then when they are quite dry break into small pieces and roast in an oven until brown. Grind as required. During the Second World War both dandelion and chicory made acceptable substitutes for coffee, but dandelion is less bitter than chicory.

Because they are so invasive, anyone wishing to cultivate dandelions for the table as a salad vegetable or cooked like spinach would be well advised to confine the seeds in boxes of rich compost; the plants can then be used as required.

Dane wort/ Dwarf elder

(Sambucus ebulus)
Family: CAPRIFOLIACEAE

Few plants have the prefix 'dane' before their common name, and those that do are often poisonous, for the Danes were a feared foe and bringers of death to small communities in Saxon England. In the seventeenth century there was even a belief that the plant grew from the blood of Danes slain by Anglo-Saxons, and in some country districts 'the danes' was a term for diarrhoea, so the Danish connotation was strong.

Another name for this small shrubby bush is 'stink wort', an apt title, for it has a very strong and most objectionable odour when the leaves and stems are crushed.

Herbal medicine enthusiasts should also be aware that dane wort is very like its cousin, common or black elder (*Sambucus nigra*), although it is a comparatively small plant, often reaching only 2m in favoured localities, but the seemingly delicious fruits are poisonous, and so is the rest of the plant. Should you accidentally gather some dane wort fruit whilst collecting elderberries for wine, the resulting brew will have a very powerful purging action. The root was used in the past as an emetic.

It was also formerly thought to induce calm and sleep, but it is far

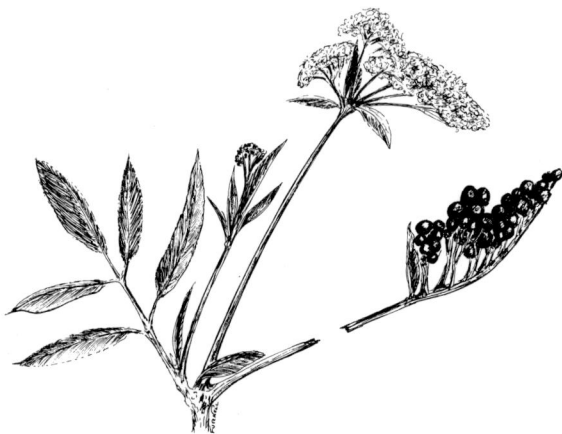

too dangerous to experiment with and is best left to skilled homoeopaths, who use an extract of the foul-smelling leaves for dropsy. The stinking leaves are also used as a poultice for boils and for treating ulcers, but there are far more pleasant remedies.

In America, a plant also known as dwarf elder (*Aralia hispida*) has many medicinal properties especially for relieving the symptoms of urinary and kidney complaints.

Dog rose

(Rosa canina)
Family: ROSACEAE

Roses are referred to in much of our literature; Shakespeare especially adopted them as symbols in many of his plays. Our modern domesticated rose owes its vigour to the wild briar form, for it is now usual to graft tender species of ornamental roses on to a wild rootstock.

It is thought the name 'dog rose' originates from the same source as many wild plants considered of little use to man, whereas ornamental roses are thought to derive from plants brought to England from Persia (Iran) as spoils of the Crusaders, although there were roses in British gardens long before that.

Rosa canina will sometimes produce sports with double flowers, and variations in colour run from pure white with an almost porcelain quality to a deep pink.

Medicinally, rose leaves or flowers have very little to offer, but the root is said to have been employed in Saxon times to ease the pain of wolf bites. In fact, there are few recorded instances of men being attacked by wolves, and many of these can be dismissed as fanciful, or were caused by carelessness, with a wolf retaliating whilst being captured for wolf baiting, or when trapped by a snare or gin trap.

There are also stories of roots being prescribed for treating bites caused by mad dogs, and this could have led to the name dog rose, but it seems unlikely.

The term 'dog' was certainly meant in a derogatory fashion, yet the plant does possess medicinal powers. Oddly enough, it was not until just prior to the Second World War that the seed cases of the rose hip were found to contain one of the most abundant sources of vitamin C in the plant kingdom. Schemes to gather hips and extract the vitamin abounded, and many senior citizens will remember the rations of rose hip syrup that ensured their children's health during the war.

The seed case contains the vitamin; the seeds themselves have little medicinal virtue, although the irritating silky down that fills the spaces between seeds and seed case has been used in France and Eastern Europe as a worm treatment, with whole rose hips being made into jam. It works by mechanical rather than chemical action, and the additional virtue of vitamins and minerals improved overall health.

Nowadays commercially produced vitamin C (ascorbic acid) has made the natural product commercially redundant, but rose hip jam, jelly and syrup will always have a place in the natural medicine chest.

The tissue-paper-like petals of dog roses and commercially developed ornamental roses can be prepared as rose water by steeping fresh rose petals in distilled water for 24 hours. This makes a good skin-toning lotion. Both rose water and oil of roses are commercially available from many pharmacists and herbal stockists.

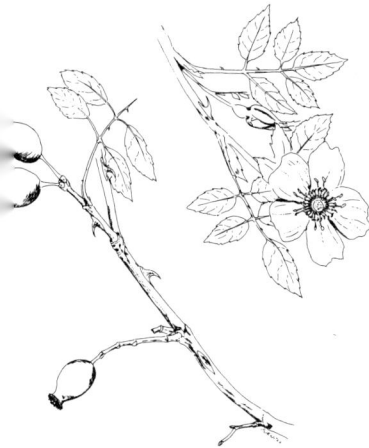

Elder
(Sambucus nigra)
Family: CAPRIFOLIACEAE

USA: known as European elder but does not occur in USA. The USA species is sweet elder (*Sambucus canadensis*)

It is hard to believe that elder trees are relatives of the fragrant honeysuckle. Elder flowers don't have the delicate scent of wild woodbine, but what they lack in perfume they make up in versatility.

In 1644 a herbalist called Martin Blockwich wrote a 200-page treatise on the elder called *Anatomie of the Elder*. In it he listed over seventy different illnesses for which elder was said to be of value in treatment or cure. And the sage and diarist John Evelyn wrote that if the medicinal properties of elder's bark, root and leaves were fully known, countrymen could find a cure for all their ills from the hedgerow. There is no doubt that elder has been a valued part of the herbalist's collection for thousands of years.

Elder has fourteen names in common use in England, ranging from 'bore tree' to 'tea tree' and 'devil's wood'. The name 'elder' has its roots in the past and was very likely derived from the Anglo-Saxon *ellarn*, meaning to kindle a fire; this could have come from the fact that hollow elder stems were used to blow a fire into life, and when dried the pith from the stems made good tinder.

Even its scientific generic name has its origins in history. It is thought that the Greek musical instrument called a *sambuke* was originally made from elder wood, and there is some verification here in that even today Italians carve a simple wind instrument called a *sampogna* from elder wood.

Because the timber is light and tough, skewers and shoemakers' pegs were made from it, and it was strong enough to be used by weavers for needles.

It's hard to say whether elder was more popular as a dye than as a medicinal herb, but there are records of Romans using the berries as hair colouring, and if ripe berries are steeped overnight in boiling water they will give a lustrous blue-black dye. However, if you contemplate trying this, be warned that the dye is just as effective on your scalp as on your hair. Used as a tint, though, it gives hair a glowing look. The leaves produce a green dye and the bark a black one for woollen fabrics, but it tends to fade rather quickly and needs to be blended with other, stronger pigments to give permanency.

A very popular application of the berries and flower heads is as a medicine for uplifting the spirit. I mean, of course, elderberry/flower wine. Elderberries make excellent wine, and in the past have been used to adulterate cheap imported grape wine to improve its flavour and give it body. There are as many recipes for elderberry and elderflower wines as there are days in the month, but an important thing to bear in mind is that the unripe berries contain a poison similar to prussic acid which can produce flushing and hot rashes in some people.

Eaten raw, the ripe fruit is considered an excellent laxative, and fresh shoots, boiled before they

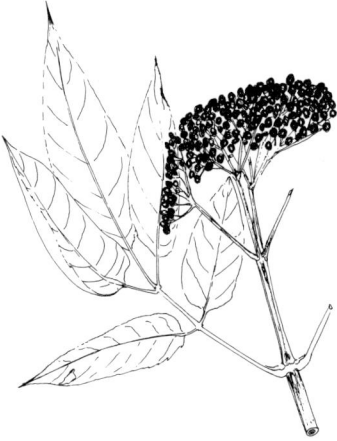

have had time to toughen up, are said to be a good decongestant for stubborn coughs.

The frothy creamy white umbels of elder flowers are looked upon by herbalists, both past and present, as a potent source of remedies promoting perspiration and lowering temperatures, often a frequent symptom of the common cold. An infusion of dried elder flowers in hot water is also recommended for reducing the discomfort of sinusitis and nasal catarrh.

Leaves and flowers can be made into a lotion which has valuable antiseptic properties and was applied in the past as a remedy for skin infections and to wash varicose ulcers. The leaves, which give off an unpleasant smell when crushed, are good as a skin dressing to keep off biting insects. However, the alkaloid sambucine present in the leaves can cause a reaction on sensitive skin and

before any lotions or dressings derived from plants are used they should be applied to a small area first as a check. Should a reaction occur then the lotion must be discarded.

Elders are also known as 'badger's herbs', for they are very often found growing near ancient badger setts, and it is not uncommon to see large elder bushes, almost reaching tree proportions, where badgers have provided fertile conditions for their growth. It is possible that the badgers use elder's insect-repellent leaves as a bedding material to keep skin parasites at bay.

Elecampane
(Inula helenium)
Family: COMPOSITAE

USA: elecampane, horse heal, yellow starwort

Elecampane is as beautiful as it is medicinally effective. Also known as wild sunflower, it is a member of the same family. Its Latin name derives from a supposed connection with the legendary Helen of Troy, but the connection is tenuous, to say the least. As she was carried off by Paris it is said that she held in her hands a bunch of elecampane.

It is also called 'horse elder', which could be a corruption of 'horse alder', as it is often found growing wild near water, particularly streams and marshes, as do

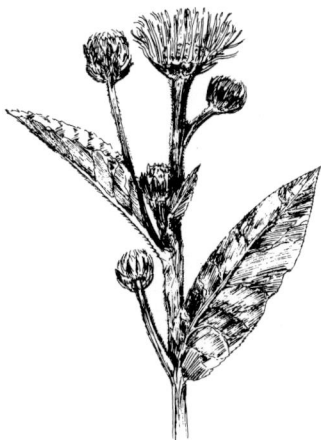

alder trees. It is known that elecampane roots were used in poultices by horse doctors in the early Victorian era for relieving saddle- and harness-sores, a malady all too common among overworked and neglected cab or hire horses.

It is likely that Roman settlers brought the plant with them to the British Isles, but it is now rare in the countryside, being mainly a garden escapee appearing on wasteland or municipal rubbish tips in country areas. It grows best in fertile, warm soil.

'Scabwort' was another of its country names, and a similar Continental member of this family (*Inula viscosa*) was used in Italy and southern France as a fly paper. The stems and leaves are sticky and were hung up in the evening so flies would roost overnight and so become stuck to the foliage. It must have been effective, for this method is still used in Europe, although not in Britain or the USA, as far as I know.

Wild elecampane is a tall majestic plant with a cluster of daisy-like yellow or orange flowers at the top of a stout hairy stem. However, despite all the foliage, it is mainly the root that is used medicinally, particularly for stomach disorders and the relief of bronchitis. It makes a potent brew, especially when mixed with coltsfoot, another member of the family compositae.

Elecampane root is large and hard, described in some herbals as horn-like in consistency, and when grown in favourable situations the root system is often quite bulky, weighing several pounds. The hard brown outer covering is scraped or peeled away and the pale inner root grated or crushed to a paste. It is most commonly used in an infusion. 50g of dried crushed root to 1 litre of water should be brought to the boil for about 10 minutes then allowed to cool. When it is strained, 1 cupful per day is the recommended dose for mild gastric disorders and general stomach upsets. The French thought it a good remedy for stomach pains suffered by young girls prior to puberty and in Roman herbals it is listed as being effective for regularizing menstruation in young women. It has a bitter flavour, even though it contains the substance inulin (diabetic sugar) and also an aromatic oil with the faintest odour of violets.

Elecampane is not only effective when taken internally. A stronger brew of 50g of root to $\frac{1}{2}$ litre of water used to be a popular treatment for skin disorders. Herbalists ancient and modern have considered it one of the best herbal remedies for irritation caused by the herpes virus. It has no measured effect on the virus itself, but the dry scabby eruptions that sometimes follow herpes infection are greatly helped by an application of infused root.

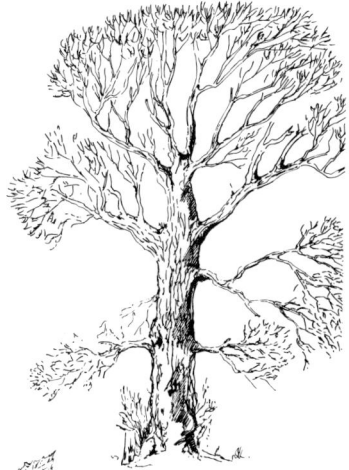

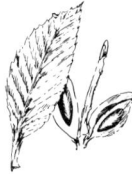

Elm
(Ulmus campestris)
Family: ULMACEAE

When the rather small unassuming beetle scolitis carried the dreaded Dutch elm disease to hedgerow giants in Great Britain it not only wiped out a feature of the English countryside that had been the subject of artists and writers for centuries, in one fell swoop it also destroyed a veritable medicine chest of benefits to mankind.

Elms have featured in the life of man for thousands of years. The beautiful wood is almost unsurpassed as a furnishing timber and is very tough, frequently being used as the basis of axleblocks and cart bearings.

There's an old wives' tale that elm makes poor firewood, being slow to burn. I suspect this is a story put about by woodmen of old so they wouldn't be given the job of splitting elm logs for the fire – a rather heavy and thankless task. Indeed, when dry the wood burns with great heat and is long-lasting.

Elm branches are often shed by the tree in times of drought, and these used to be converted into the finest medicinal charcoal, administered to reduce flatulence caused by impoverished diet and intestinal worms. Ground charcoal of both elm and beech, when mixed with an oil of male fern (*Dryopteris filix-mas*) was formerly prescribed to rid the intestines of tapeworms and roundworms. Today worms are rarely heard of, since they mainly affect people dealing with domesticated farm animals, and modern worm tablets are so effective as to have rendered elm charcoal and male fern remedy redundant.

The elm played its part in treating other digestive ailments, too. The inner bark, sweet-tasting with a high level of minerals and nutrients, was prepared as a floury gruel to be taken for intestinal infections and diarrhoea.

The outer bark was used in the preparation of leather. The lighter colour of skins tanned with elm is distinct from those tanned with oak, and they were popular with wealthy merchants.

Elm leaves, too, were beneficial for skin infections, and crushed leaves applied as a poultice healed grazes and could be adapted as an emergency dressing. The leaves contain considerable quantities of tannin, and a mucilage that forms a skin over wounds, so helping to prevent infection. Modern man has such a high level of overall health that a festering wound is almost unheard-of today, but to our forefathers a cut or bad graze could very easily lead to severe skin infection, temporary disability and loss of earnings.

The leaf galls of elm leaves are full of an oily fluid produced by the tree to reduce depredations by the gall wasp. This liquid was once thought to be a perfect cosmetic for improving complexions; it also makes an effective wound dressing, though difficult to gather.

Powdered bark of the American slippery elm (*Ulmus fulva*) was used by American Indians for stomach ailments, and when mixed with honey it's quite a nourishing and valuable food. European settlers who sowed their own species of elm for similar purposes found that slippery elm supplied an efficient medicine for easing colitis and infections of the digestive system. It was prescribed as a remedy for gastric and peptic ulcers, but recent medicinal advances have led to a decline in its popularity in conventional medical circles, though it's still widely used by herbalists.

A mixture of slippery elm bark powder and powdered charcoal applied to a boil as a hot poultice still has its devotees.

Evening primrose
(Oenothera biennis)
Family: ONAGRACEAE

Tracing the origins of evening primrose is a difficult business. It appears to have been introduced to the American continent from Europe in the sixteenth century as a root vegetable, then reintroduced into Britain much later. It does grow wild in Britain, but only because it once escaped from someone's garden, and appears to thrive only where the climate is softer, as in the west of England.

A tall, elegant plant, it has large papery flowers of a soft yellow. These attract night-flying moths which pollinate the plant. Its

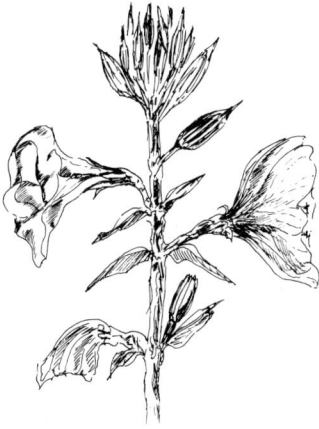

flowering period is long, as each spike supports lots of flowers, and the spike can grow up to 2m tall in favourable conditions.

It is biennial, and in the first season all growth goes into producing an edible fleshy root, not unlike parsnip. This and the young leaves have made it a popular natural food, especially in parts of America where it is known as wild beet.

Recently new processes have been developed to extract the oil, which is rich in a substance also found in sunflower seeds, called gamma-linolenic acid. It is believed that this substance will strengthen the body's own biochemical processes. However, there are many problems in producing the oil in commercially economic quantities, and at present it is very expensive to extract and refine, but if you wish to grow the plant yourself for its edible roots and foliage and beautiful soft-yellow sweetly scented flowers, you will not go unrewarded.

Feverfew
(Chrysanthemum parthenium)
Family: COMPOSITAE

This small, rather fragrant member of the daisy family ranks very high on lists of medicinal herbs, and has been in use since ancient Greek times. Indeed, the latter part of its scientific name is supposed to refer to an incident in Greek history when a man who had fallen from the Parthenon during its construction was cured of his head injuries by treatment based on feverfew.

The origin of the name 'feverfew' is difficult to trace, but it may have been derived from the old English *feferfuge*, coming from the Latin word *febrifugia*, or it may have less ancient origins. In the Middle Ages it was called 'featherfoil' or 'feather leaf', for the leaves are feathery.

Medicinally, feverfew was highly valued for relieving ague, the old term for malaria, a sickness endemic in these islands until the fens of East Anglia were drained. As well as ague, it was used to relieve symptoms of giddiness and vertigo, and also for head stuffiness following a cold. There is good reason to connect the two, for giddiness and vertigo associated with inner ear infections are sometimes after-effects of a cold.

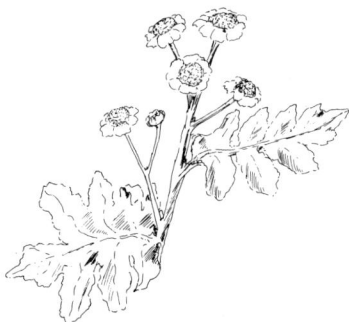

Our forefathers were great ones for a cure-all, and when a plant proved valuable for one ailment it was often added to the general armoury and attributed with powers it did not actually possess. For instance, as well as being a specific for colds, dizziness and chest infections, feverfew was recommended for suppressing urine and promoting the menstrual cycle when it had been delayed for some reason or other. It was generally assumed that this herb had the power to procure an abortion in the very early weeks of pregnancy, but there is no evidence to support this, although to be absolutely sure, it should be avoided in pregnancy.

It was taken in an infusion to clear the kidneys of ill humours, to expel worms, and as a tonic, and there are interesting references in some herbals to feverfew as a medicine to help opium addicts over the trauma of an overdose. Apart from the general tonic abilities of this plant, none of the fanciful claims made on its behalf appear to have any foundation in fact.

However, more recently feverfew has sprung to prominence as a cure for migraine headaches, or more accurately, as a preventative measure to avoid headache developing in the first place. There are many who swear by the fact that one leaf every day in a sandwich stops their migraine, or at least reduces the frequency and severity of attacks. (It should always be taken in this way, as otherwise it can cause mouth ulcers.)

Research into feverfew and migraine is currently being carried out in Britain, the United States and Europe, although so far results are inconclusive. Nevertheless, if you suffer from this affliction and wish to experiment with feverfew, the best course of action is to eat one small fresh leaf of feverfew in a sandwich every day for a full calendar month, noting the frequency of migraine attacks. Then refrain from taking any for another full calendar month, again checking the frequency of attacks. You will then be able to tell if the herb has had any effect.

It seems that feverfew will work for some people where others gain no benefit at all. The herb is harmless in small quantities and well worth trying.

Fig
(Ficus carica)
Family: MORACAE

It is fitting that the leaf Adam and Eve chose to cover their nakedness in the Garden of Eden after they had transgressed through disobeying the word of God was a fig leaf, for figs have been associated with man for as long as civilization itself.

Although fig trees are not at home in Great Britain, they will fruit and ripen into an edible state, especially in gardens in the west of England.

At the end of the Edwardian era, figs fell into some disrepute through overuse of syrup of figs to regularize bowel movements — even when they didn't need to be regularized. But to dismiss figs as merely a laxative is to do them immense disservice, for in the past this tree has often induced men to fight wars over land where fig trees would thrive and bear fruit.

Primitive man was a hunter-gatherer, who learned to glean a living from the countryside. Even before they domesticated cattle and sheep, and learned to raise grain for food, primitive peoples had already realized that dried figs were an easily stored source of energy and that fresh figs provided not only food, but vital minerals and vitamins to keep them healthy.

The Middle East, still the best place for cultivating figs, held the key to many medicinal recipes for this delicious fruit and the leaves and sap that flow from freshly cut stems. Egyptians venerated fig trees, and adopted them for medicines and for ceremonials to their dead. In the Book of Isaiah were used to save a king from what is described as a serious tumour. King Hezekiah of Judah was sick unto death when the prophet Isaiah told them to lay figs on him as a dressing and the king recovered. It is likely the problem was a serious abcess or carbuncle that was endangering his life.

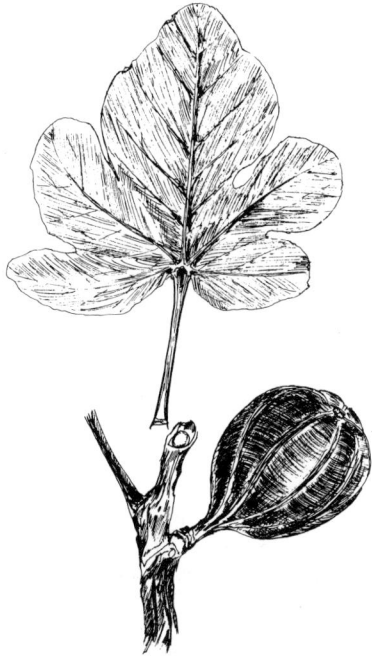

Among other properties figs contain a lot of sugar, especially when dried. Sugar is well known as a fungicide and bactericide when found in sufficient concentrations, and so there would be considerable benefit in a poultice of dried figs. The sugar would also absorb some of the moisture from a bad infection.

The sugar with which figs are so well endowed must have played havoc with people's teeth, yet they were recommended by the Hebrews as a remedy for gum disorders and mouth ulcers.

The Greeks placed it higher even than the middle-eastern civilizations did, for they considered the fig to be food for the mind. Plato called it the 'philosopher's friend', because it was supposed to strengthen intelligence, and mixed together in a paste with hazelnuts it was prescribed as a proof against poisoning, a fairly common hazard in Ancient Greece, especially for philosophers and senators.

The founders of Rome, the twins Romulus and Remus, were said to have been abandoned under a fig tree before the she-wolf found and suckled them, and the Romans revered figs every bit as much as the Greeks. Cultivation of the fruit was perfected by them, and they prized its food value. Its property as a laxative has been acknowledged for centuries and has sound basis in fact, for the seeds stimulate bowel movements and the fruit capsules in which the seeds are contained are a valuable source of roughage. Yet it is as a cough remedy that they are best docu-mented. Six figs can be boiled in milk for 10 minutes, and a cupful of this liquid taken several times a day.

Another recipe for a cough is to roast six figs in the oven until they are dry enough to be ground to a powder. This powder can be made into a drink rather like coffee as and when required, and the same powder mixed with honey is said to be good for relieving itching chilblains.

Fresh fig leaves made into a tea are good for relieving coughs, and where the leaf is pulled the sap that oozes from the wound is said to remove warts and corns. It seems there's not much for which figs cannot be used.

Flax
(Linum usitatissimum)
Family: LINACEAE

In the latter half of the nineteenth century there was a thriving industry fuelled by flax. It was grown for fibre and for linseed oil, and in meadows and valleys it bloomed bright cornflower-blue in the early summer sunshine.

Common flax is one of the oldest known cultivated plants; it is doubtful if there is any such thing as a truly wild flax plant. It grows well in the mild climate of the British Isles, and even today there is an industry in Ireland based on flax and the linen derived from its fibrous stems.

Remnants of linen have been

linen. Linseed oil is the basis for many industrial products, from paint to cattle food. The seeds, brown and glossy, contain a rich oil, and it is on this oil that the paint industry was based, although nowadays many of the oils used in manufacturing paint are synthetic.

Linoleum, the standard floor covering until ousted by harder-wearing plastic materials, was made from linseed oil together with a variety of fillers and pigments.

Just beneath the seed case there is a plentiful supply of mucilage which has value as a laxative and lubricant to the intestines. Linseed oil refined by boiling has similar properties, and it is as a remedy for digestive ailments that linseed itself is recommended.

However, some herbal practitioners are less than enthusiastic about using raw seeds in any remedy, and in any case they should be soaked in water overnight. For indigestion you can make up a mixture of seeds with liquorice and honey to mask the otherwise unpleasant taste. A teaspoonful of seeds (soaked overnight) is mixed with a teaspoon of liquorice in $\frac{1}{2}$ litre of boiling water. Allow to stand for ten minutes, then strain and sweeten with honey. This should be taken on an empty stomach.

For thousands of years linseed oil has been applied to prepare wood for hard usage, and its property of reducing dryness and pro-

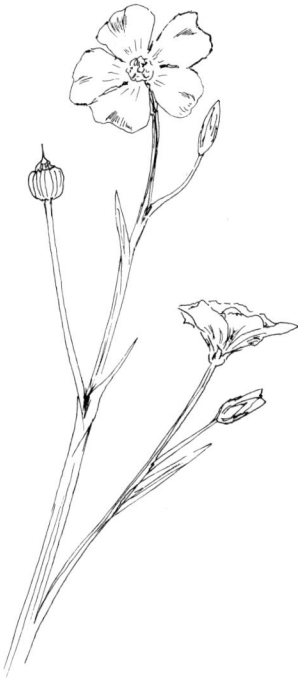

found in ancient burials, and it is known that when the Egyptians wove flax fibres all those centuries ago the skills they employed in weaving and dressing the fibres had already been in use for several thousand years.

For a fibre to remain popular through so many centuries it must provide outstanding comfort and hard-wearing features, and this is just what flax and its linen fibres possess.

As if the property to yield linen were not enough, linseed from ripe flax seedpods has supported an industry almost as important as

tecting the grain most likely led to its use by workmen to treat work-hardened hands and cracked skin, and later as a poultice for abcesses and infected cuts. The seeds themselves are crushed to a meal and employed in the preparation of poultices and lotions. It's best to do this yourself to make sure the meal is fresh, as fermentation of a poultice kept too long produces prussic acid, which can itself cause inflammation.

A tablespoonful of crushed seed is made into a paste with a little boiling water. Add this paste to a litre of boiling water, and continue to boil for two minutes. This can be put into bath water to soften the skin and reduce dryness. It's also said to have a sedative effect. This same paste can be applied as a poultice for boils and skin eruptions, but it should not be boiled. Spread it on a hot cloth, place over the boil and change frequently.

It is also said to be a very soothing remedy for muscle pain and sprains, and it's comfortable to use, for it is applied only warm, not very hot as is usual with poultices. The secret of linseed lies in its preparation and freshness.

Fleabane

(Pulicaria dysenterica)
Family: COMPOSITAE

USA: horseweed

It is only in relatively recent times that Western man has been free

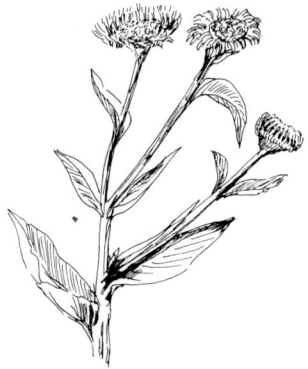

from the attentions of external parasites. Some, like fleas, are still subject to periodic eruptions in numbers, as older properties are refurbished, with central heating installed and fitted carpets laid on loose boarded floors. This creates a heaven on earth for the human flea and its close relative the cat flea, both of which need quiet undisturbed dusty warmth as provided by a closely carpeted corner in which to lay their eggs and allow their larvae to reach maturity.

Inspection of medieval literature, Shakespeare's plays and the writings of Chaucer show that fleas were part of everyday life for our forefathers and something that everyone, from the highest to the lowest, had to bear. Fleabites were just as likely in the king's feather-down bed as in the straw-filled pallets of the meanest of his subjects. In summer, when the activities of these creatures were at their height, life must have been intolerable.

Fleas who plunged their mouthparts into the skins of sixteenth- and seventeenth-century sleepers had often enjoyed their last meal on the blood of a plague-carrying black rat, which heralded a more sinister outcome than mere irritation. As well as the dreaded Black Death, bubonic plague, fleas carried a host of other diseases and could even transmit malaria under certain circumstances, for although this disease is considered to be sub-tropical, it was endemic in England under the name ague until the 1850s.

It was the sheer debilitating effects of constant flea attacks which led herbalists to turn their ingenuity to seeking a deterrent to fleas. To aid them they used members of the daisy family, especially common fleabane. It is actually recorded that when strewn in sleeping quarters this plant acted as a deterrent to the fleas' activities. There is also proof that juice extracted from the flowers and leaves and refined will have a deleterious effect on these insects.

Extracts of plants from the compositae family have insecticidal properties. However, as well as being a well-tried deterrent to insect pests, fleabane was treasured for its effect on the digestive tract, especially when epidemics of dysentry swept the land, and was used distilled for treating diarrhoea.

In the seventeenth century a fleabane was imported from the Americas which was much used by North American Indians for treating digestive tract infections. It was called *Erigeron canadense* and is related to our native blue fleabane *Erigeron acre*, but with stronger properties. When distilled, the volatile oil of erigeron is obtained, which is used as a diuretic to treat kidney disorders and for soothing sore throats, especially tonsillitis.

Common fleabane (*Pulicaria dysenterica*) is prepared as a tea by steeping 2 tablespoonfuls of whole dried plant in 1 litre of boiling water for 10 minutes. Then strain and give the patient 2 dessertspoonfuls to ease discomfort. It's extremely astringent and bitter to taste, and this astringent property was used to reduce bleeding from uterine infections before other, safer methods were devised.

It is a common plant of alkaline soils, found in mid-July growing on roadside banks and in field margins, and is much visited by smaller butterflies and moths.

Fumitory
(Fumaria officinalis)
Family: PAPAVERACEAE

USA: American, or Indian, fumitory (*Fumaria indica*)

Not so very long ago there was a time when the acquisition of a suntan was considered highly undesirable. Indeed, many a lady in Georgian or Victorian England would have been most upset by the effects of the sun on her skin.

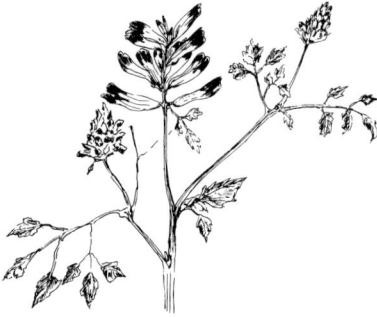

In those days it was usual for wives and daughters of the gentry to wear outdoor clothes which ensured that the health-giving rays of the sun never came anywhere near their complexions. It was fashionable to be pale and interesting. How they coped with the effects of vitamin D deficiency is not documented, but the general health of ladies in those days was often far from good. Perhaps the custom for women to stay closeted indoors contributed to the spread of the dread disease, consumption, known to us as tuberculosis.

Peasants in the field and dairymaids in the byre were equally susceptible to disease, but in their case the susceptibility was often caused by lack of proper food and sheer grinding hard labour. At least there was no shortage of sunlight-induced vitamin D, but vanity is classless and the village maids strove to emulate their pale-faced 'betters' by bleaching the roses from their cheeks with a variety of mixtures. Some of these were noxious, but others, like

fumitory, when boiled in milk could be pleasant and soothing to the skin.

We are not sure how this delicate plant got its name but one school of thought has suggested that it came from the plant's appearance: rather like smoke wreathing up from the regions of darkness. Fumitory juice is irritant, and was used in the past to clear the eyes; perhaps its ability to bring on tears was likened to the effect of smoke in the eyes.

Whatever the derivation of its name, there is little doubt that our forefathers ranked fumitory high on the list of medicinal herbs. It was used for liver disorders, especially jaundice, and for digestive problems and urine retention. An infusion of fumitory was recommended for eczema and skin troubles. In short, it was a general tonic.

Many of the ills which have afflicted civilized man have been self-induced, partly by the types of food consumed. 'We are what we eat' is a good saying, and just as modern ills of circulatory diseases and carcinoma are as much a part of the twentieth century as the motor car and television, so liver and digestive ills were the lot of pre-technological man.

When fumitory was used to relieve jaundice it was noticed that, as the treatment progressed and patients recovered, the stimulant effect was reversed, reducing circulation and acting more like a sedative in causing patients to become calm and drowsy. Because of this it was recommended that preparations containing fumitory should not be used for more than eight consecutive days. If a patient was being treated for removal of bodily toxins, a break of an equal number of days before resuming treatment was the rule. However, if fumitory was to be used as a sedative, then the effect would be progressive, from eight to twenty days. All very complicated, and not at all like the simple lotion that peasant girls used to whiten their skin.

Modern drugs have replaced fumitory in treating liver disorders, so its value as a constituent in skin lotions can be further explored. 60g of whole plant should be boiled in $\frac{1}{2}$ litre of milk; this can be used either as a compress or as a lotion. The solution will not keep for more than a few days even in a refrigerator, but when fresh it can be extremely efficacious for dry and flaking skin. One word of warning here. Don't use it in milk for eczema, for in many cases this condition is the manifestation of an allergy to dairy products.

It is probably best not to pick those plants growing by the wayside, for as with many herbs near busy roads they take up heavy metals, such as lead, in their foliage, with detrimental results. Medicinal or cosmetic herbs should be picked only from a well-known unpolluted site or purchased from a reputable supplier. Fumitory is a common plant and can be gathered all through summer, although it's at its best in June when the pink-and-white flowers with their distinctive purple tips are just opening. It should be dried in the shade as quickly as possible to retain its properties; an airing cupboard is ideal.

Garlic
(Allium sativum)
Family: LILIACEAE

Garlic seems to arouse almost more interest than any other medicinal herb and because it grows very well under cultivation it deserves a special mention.

Not without reason, it is known as an outlaw of the lily family. Its pungent after-smell on the breath has stopped more than one budding romance in its tracks. 'Garlic is for two' should be the motto of the Garlic Producers' Federation, were such an organization to exist, for to eat garlic alone is to know true ostracism. It is said that if you rub the soles of your feet with a cut clove of garlic the smell will be on your breath within the hour. I've never had the courage to try it!

Wild garlic grows in a number of countries in the northern hemisphere, and recently, while reading an American book on herbs called *Eat the Weeds*, now, sadly, out of print, I discovered that American Huron Indians used it in soup and considered it extremely valuable as a medicinal herb.

The American Indians were very skilled and knowledgeable about medicinal plants, and in an epic journey undertaken through the untamed wilds of that continent in 1674, beginning from Green Bay and finishing up on the shores of the Great Lakes at what was later to become Chicago, the explorer Marquette recorded that they survived the journey by eating large quantities of garlic bulbs. Under the circumstances they would have had little trouble from the natives, and the vitamin and mineral content of garlic would certainly have helped to keep away diseases such as scurvy, for garlic is an excellent source of vitamin C when eaten in large quantities. It also contains reasonable quantities of vitamins A and B and active minerals such as sulphur and iron, as well as calcium.

The plant has a long illustrious history and in the Talmud it is stated that garlic kept the body warm, brightened the face and fostered love – and as if that were not enough, it killed parasites and jealousy.

The Egyptians revered it. The Romans gave it to their workmen and soldiers. To the former it was said to impart strength and in the latter it excited courage. Game cocks were made more aggressive by a diet of garlic before a fight.

In medicine its uses are more prosaic, but there are regular references to its being prescribed to reduce infestations of intestinal parasites, and indeed it was frequently used as a panacea for worms in children in country districts in Europe well into this century.

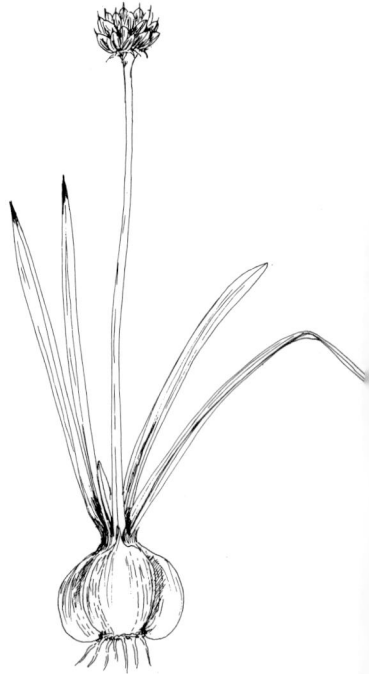

The Irish, who live in a climate more conducive to lung infections than most, have employed garlic for three or four hundred years in cough syrups, and it also played a part in so-called 'elixirs of youth'. In pre-Second World War Bulgaria, peasants in the mountains were living to great ages still in good health and vigour on a simple diet that contained a high proportion of garlic. However, it is likely that their relatively stress-free existence in the healthy mountain air played a greater part in this than did the pungent bulb.

Nowadays garlic is primarily a culinary herb, and a much valued one at that. Nevertheless, there are more properties in this herb than you may imagine, and for those who would like to partake but can't stand the smell there are now odour-free garlic extracts accredited with equal power.

Ginger
(Zingiber officinale)
Family: ZINGIBERACEAE

Certain plants are known to be of Chinese origin, and consequently their use either for culinary or medicinal purposes is very well documented. Ginger is a good example, for the Chinese have employed the root as a medicine and a condiment for several thousand years; indeed, they exported it via the silk route to Mediterranean cultures.

Ancient Greeks wrote about it, including Dioscorides who recommended it for cooking and as a stomach-calming agent.

Ginger root is the part of greatest value. In the natural state a reed-like stem grows from the thickened rhizome-like structure. When gathered, the root is dried and powdered and stored in tightly closed containers to keep its active principles intact. All over the East ginger is regarded as a beneficial herb, mainly because of its valued place in proprietary curry powders, where its quality of enhancing flavour whilst assisting digestion is greatly treasured.

Chinese herbalists employed ginger in medicines to relieve gastric imbalance and flatulence, and some cooks actually chewed the root to reduce the feeling of nausea

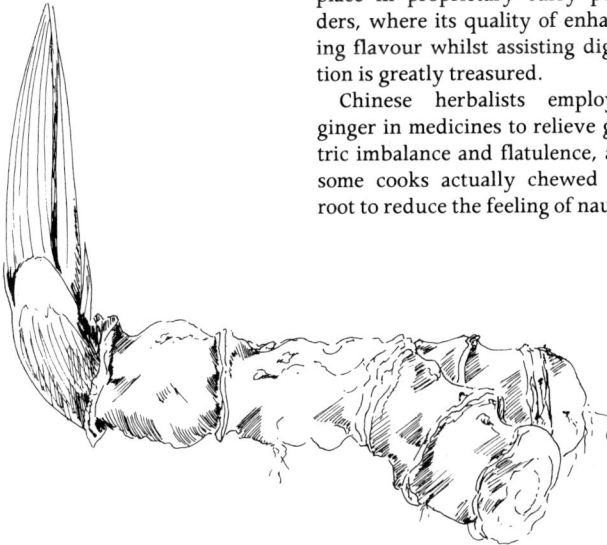

caused by being exposed to cooking fumes all day.

The power of this plant to act upon the sympathetic nervous system has long been known by sailors of the East, where ginger powder is prescribed to keep seasickness at bay during long voyages across the stormy China Sea. Chinese pirates adopted it for this purpose and recently American marines have carried out a study into various types of anti-motion-sickness remedies including ginger. Results of these tests, together with a previous test on students, indicates that people who had been given a standard dose of 940g of dried ginger root in water were able to withstand the effects of rotation in a special chair for two to three times longer than a control group who had been given a harmless placebo or a proprietary travel-sickness drug.

Research continues in the United States into the value of ginger as an anti-motion-sickness treatment, but crystallized ginger taken by my own family on our small boat has proved quite effective; there is no doubt that ginger does have a calming quality on the balance organs, and the discomfort caused by motion sickness can be considerably allayed.

Needless to say, there is one proviso; little measurable result will be felt if ginger is taken to relieve symptoms already existing. It's valid only if taken as a preventative measure before undertaking a journey. Relief is maintained by eating small pieces of ginger, which appear to allow the body to cope with the unfamiliar and disquieting action of waves.

As a remedy for dyspepsia, mix 900g of dried ginger root with $\frac{1}{4}$ litre of boiling water. This does have a rather fiery taste, but it can be modified by adding a teaspoonful of honey, and a similar brew using twice the quantity of ginger to the same amount of water is recommended for lessening the discomfort of menstrual periods in very cold weather.

Ginger tea is sometimes used as a hangover remedy because of its calming properties and ability to reduce nausea, so allowing the body to recover from alcohol excess.

Ginseng
(*Panax schinseng* – Asian, *Panax quinquefolius* – American)
Family: ARALIACEA

The root of this long-lived, slow-maturing plant grows in mountain forest areas in China and Asia, where its delicate foliage pushes up into the soft woodland light. It is an odd plant and at one time was thought impossible to cultivate under artificial conditions, but now it is grown in many countries as a cash crop, albeit on a small scale.

It prefers deep shade and will soon fail in bright sunlight so it can

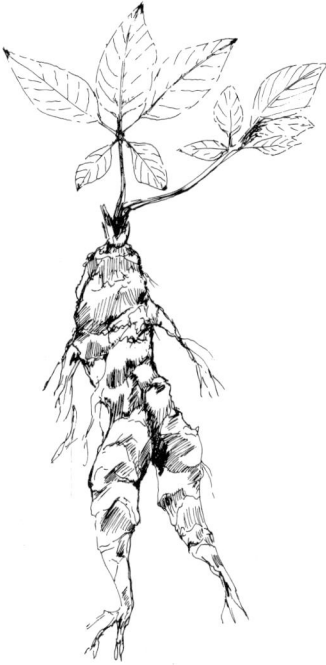

many problems from painful joints to high blood pressure, allows concentration to be unimpaired after periods of prolonged effort and gives a feeling of general well-being.

The Chinese are masters of herbal medicine, and the 'barefoot doctors' have recourse to ginseng for a multitude of purposes. The name 'ginseng' is said to be an anglicized version of the Chinese word for 'man plant', which came about because, as well as being a panacea for all ills, the root is said to resemble the shape of a man's body, and appears to be treated in the East with the same superstitious awe as was the mandrake root during the Middle Ages in Europe.

In China ginseng is used to promote well-being even in those who enjoy good health, and also to prolong life, and Eastern political leaders have attributed their active old age to regular use of this magic root.

There are many different stories about the merits of ginseng, depending on the country of origin. Korean ginseng is attributed with a finer quality, but the Chinese product is said to be more potent. Indeed, in China it is known as 'the golden one', not because of its colour – which is actually an overall green, the root being parsnip colour – but for the value of a mature root, which can be anything up to ten years of age before it's harvested.

be grown in Britain, and the quality of roots obtained from British ginseng is said to be quite good, if a little weak.

The power of the root, which is the part employed for medicinal and restorative purposes, is hard to define. Many of its devotees will tell you it possesses aphrodisiac properties, whilst others claim it will act as a catalyst to enable bodily functions to proceed with greater vigour. Yet despite exhaustive research carried out in Britain, America, and the Soviet Union, there is still no clear explanation as to why it appears to regularize

American ginseng is grown commercially in small fields with shading fences built between the rows. This is an adaption of the method of cultivation employed in Korea. The many processes required to achieve the finished product are complicated, and access to a supply of seedling stock is problematic, as availability is sporadic.

Prepared ginseng is available from health food stores and herbal suppliers, and although expensive it's a bestseller. All those who have tried it say different things about its efficacy, but the Russians, who are closer to Asian culture in their attitude to traditional medicines than we in the West, are said to have administered it to Soviet cosmonauts with beneficial effects. It is still treated with slight suspicion in the West, however, generally by the medical establishment.

Recently there have been doubts as to the value of taking ginseng for prolonged periods, as side effects have been reported when continued high doses are administered. It is best to take preparations containing this herb for no longer than two months at a time.

Good king henry
(Chenopodium bonus-henricus)
Family: CHENOPODIACEAE

Of the plants that man has domesticated for food and medicinal purposes, many have fallen from favour; one of these is good king henry, now considered a perni-

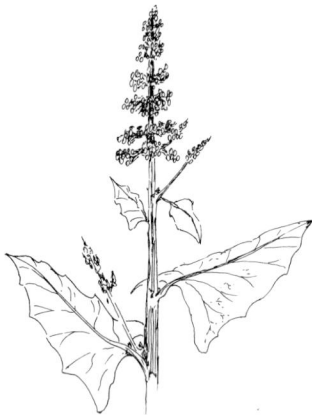

cious weed. A member of the goosefoot family, it is thought to have gained its royal name by accident rather than any connection with King Hal, being called 'good henry' to distinguish it from a similar related plant with inedible foliage called bad henry (*Malus henricus*). The word 'king' was added by medieval herbalists.

This plant has been in the service of man for thousands of years, and seeds have been found in the stomachs of Bronze Age sacrificial victims who were interred in peat bogs and have been remarkably preserved. The most famous of these victims is Tollund Man, whose leather-capped head and peaceful expression belie his death by strangulation. His last meal was porridge composed of various seeds, among them good king henry. Where other 'bog people' have been disinterred and their stomach contents examined, these same seeds were found in their digestive tracts, indicating that they were common fare for the people of those times.

In the Middle Ages it was grown as a vegetable; the stems were cut when young and the broad triangular leaves were used like spinach.

Medicinally, it was administered to relieve scurvy, as both leaves and stems contain considerable amounts of vitamin C. The plant also has iron in usable quantities, vitamin B_1, calcium and many other trace elements. It also yields valuable proteins.

Although it is considered to be an introduced plant, there is evidence to show that it has featured on the bill of fare of English peasants for centuries, and it was still cultivated until the early eighteenth century. Just at the moment it appears to be enjoying something of a renaissance as a vegetable, and garden centres can supply seeds.

As a family, the goosefoots enjoy world-wide coverage. On the American continent several species are eaten, and the Spanish conquistadors found *Chenopodium quinoa* cultivated for its edible foliage, with the seeds being ground for flour.

Another relative of good king henry, *Chenopodium anthelminticum* is used in the United States as a source of wormseed oil to expel roundworms, especially infestations in children. However, there is no record of European goosefoot

being utilized as a worm treatment. The leaves of good king henry and a related goosefoot called 'fat hen' are prepared for treating women's ailments, and Culpeper considered it excellent for all afflictions of the womb.

However, there is little to prove any direct medicinal value in this plant other than its vitamin and mineral worth and the natural fibre content which would account for references to its laxative properties in some herbals.

Great burnet
(Sanguisorba officinalis)
Family: ROSACEAE

Burnet has had a long and illustrious history as a medicinal herb, but is found growing in many herb gardens nowadays for its culinary properties rather than its medical virtues.

Great burnet is a plant of chalk soils and grows best on the lower slopes of old sheep-grazed chalk downland, now a very rare habitat in Britain.

Medicinally, burnet was used to allay bleeding and clean the horrifying wounds common in the days when weapons of war and defence were edged blades, pikes or arrows, all designed to create a large wound which caused many of the victims to die of shock and loss of blood and body fluids. Therefore any plant that could reduce bleeding, either on the battlefield or on

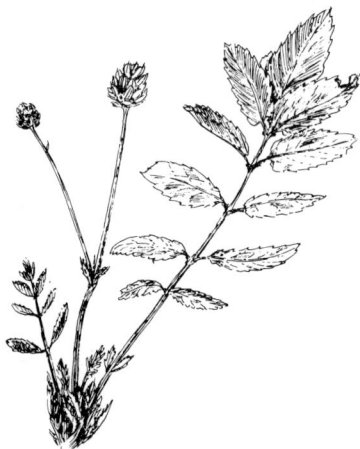

the farm, was prized, especially if it was common.

The scientific name of burnet is sanguisorba, *sanguis* being Latin for 'blood', although it was by no means the only plant with this useful property.

The closely related salad burnet (*Sanguisorba minor*) like its cousin prefers chalk soil, although salad burnet seems to thrive best on high downland proper. The flavour is similar to that of cucumber, with a hint of sharpness, and the young foliage is a useful addition to any country salad, for it has a high mineral and vitamin content, especially vitamin C.

The addition of salad burnet and greater burnet to lotions for treating mild burns, particularly sunburn, has dropped from general practice, but if you want to try it boil a handful of leaves and flowers in $\frac{1}{2}$ litre of water, strain and leave

to cool. Cool the skin by running cold water over the affected area, then cover with a poultice of crushed burnet leaves and flowers; this helps relieve any discomfort. However, this dressing is a temporary measure only and should be replaced frequently until a sterile burn dressing can be applied.

One of the main problems with burns is secondary infection, if the skin is blistered and broken. The greatest care must be taken not to keep a poultice on for too long, otherwise it may stick to the burn and break the skin.

Under no circumstances should you use burnet leaves and flowers from a pasture where horses or cattle are grazed regularly. There is always the possibility of introducing tetanus spores into an open wound, with most serious results.

However, burnet has a less dramatic role as a tonic herb and as a garnish for wine cups and drinks, where its slightly bitter taste emphasizes the flavours of other ingredients.

Ground ivy
(Glechoma hederacea)
Family: LABIATAE

USA: creeping Charlie, field balm, gill-over-the-ground, ground ivy

The bright-blue flowers of ground ivy are typical of a member of the huge labiatae family. They appear early in the year and are common over much of southern England,

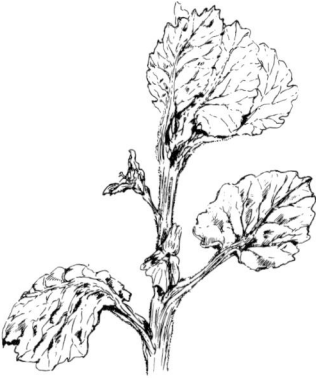

with the plant forming large mats of foliage rather in the same manner as common ivy. (This is not to be confused with poison ivy, *Rhus radicans*, more commonly found in north America.)

It has any number of common country names, from 'Gill-go-over-the-ground' to 'haymaids' and 'ale hoof'. The name 'ale hoof' is thought to have derived from its use by brewers to lengthen the keeping properties of the thin beer supplied to Royal Navy and merchantmen alike for consumption on long sea voyages.

Medicinally it has found favour as a treatment for external and internal soreness. Discomfort caused by bronchitis was eased by taking it as a syrup, and an extract in oil was applied externally.

A syrup is prepared by crushing 250g of fresh leaves and flowers in a mortar and covering with a small quantity of water. This is left to stand overnight, and the juice strained off into a cup of water.

Bring to the boil, and add sugar until the whole has a syrupy texture. Allow to cool and bottle for future use.

To produce an oil, fill a clear glass screw-topped jar with a quantity of pounded plant, then olive or sunflower oil should be added to fill any spaces. Seal and place in the sun for one month, topping up with leaf and flower as the plant material settles and adding oil to replace that which has been absorbed by the plant. After a month, strain off the oil and bottle it for future use.

Fresh ground ivy has a pleasant minty/lemony smell and this will be retained in some degree by the oil. It can be dried and kept for winter, but it flowers so early and grows so freely in the countryside that it is best used fresh.

For treating general symptoms of bronchitis, put a handful of fresh crushed plant in 1 litre of water and bring to the boil very slowly. Remove from the heat immediately on boiling, as many of this plant's active principles appear to be volatile and will be driven off by prolonged boiling. This infusion can be drunk at bedtime to promote easy breathing. The same tea is said to be soothing and calming for mucose membranes in the throat.

There are records of ground ivy being employed to treat renal colic, gallstones and general urinary infections, but there is little reason for supposing that gallstones might be affected by anything found in this plant, although it does appear to soothe some bladder inflammations and its effect on the digestive tract is well documented.

A piece of folklore connected with this plant concerns the barbaric practice of cockfighting, popular from the Middle Ages right into the early part of this century. It seems ground ivy was employed for the eye injuries often suffered by birds in the cockpit. An injured bird was treated with an application of chewed leaf, supposedly to heal the wound quickly. This practice may have come from an earlier use of an infusion of fresh ground ivy for old infected cuts, such as would result from fighting with edged weapons. An emergency plaster can be made from fresh crushed ground ivy leaves and placed over a cut to prevent infection and stem bleeding until proper treatment is obtained.

Groundsel
(Senecio vulgaris)
Family: COMPOSITAE

It would be very surprising if common groundsel were not mentioned in ancient herbals. Wherever man turns the soil, groundsel will spring up. It is extremely invasive, colonizing soil before any more heavily shading weeds can appear to oust it through competition for food and space.

It has many common names, and

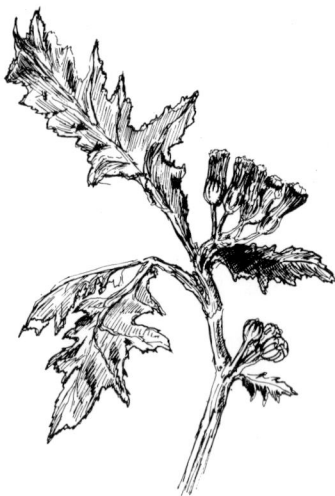

reference to the *Dictionary of English Plant Names* reveals a history reaching back to Saxon times and beyond. The Old English seventh century name is *grundeswylige*, or 'ground swallower', and refers to the ability of the prostrate leafy stems to cover ground in a very short time. A later name was *gundesuilge* and seems to refer to a use for groundsel also mentioned in later herbals, that of treating the eyes for redness and inflammation. It seems that groundsel, by whatever name, was a popular herb.

Modern gardeners would faint with shock at the prospect of cultivating groundsel, but in the Middle Ages monastery gardens would have been adequately stocked with orderly lines of groundsel plants, all awaiting their various uses. In those days, apart from its value as a constituent in

Aaron's rod *(Verbascum thapsus)*

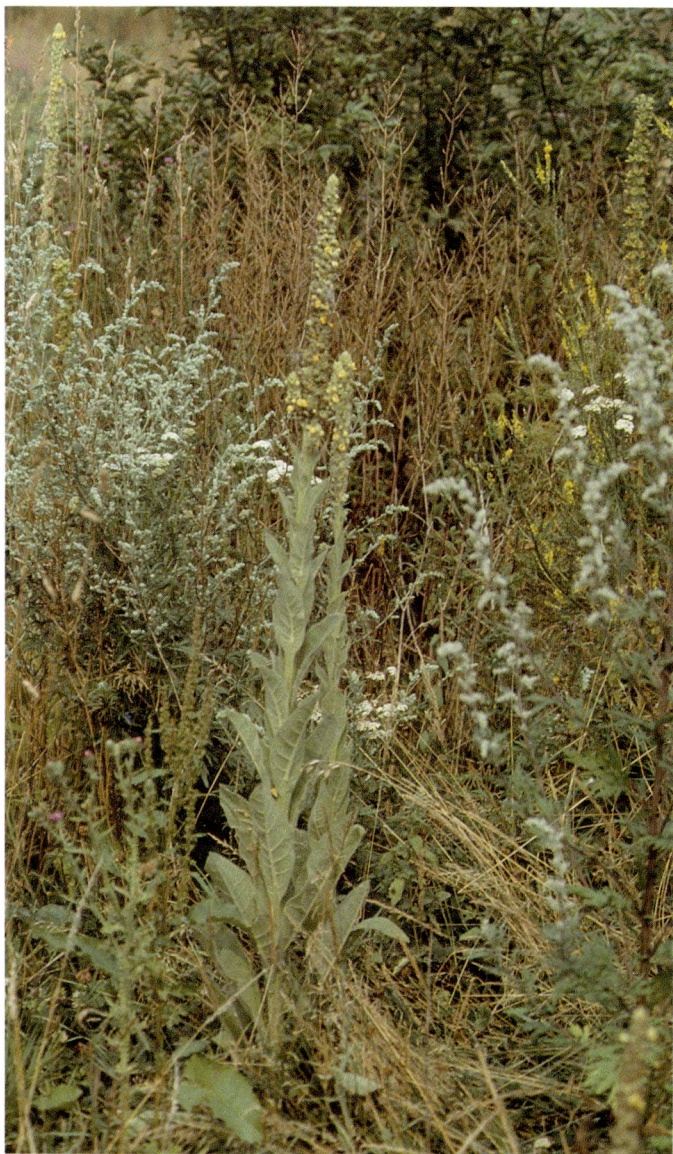

Bugle *(Ajuga reptans)*

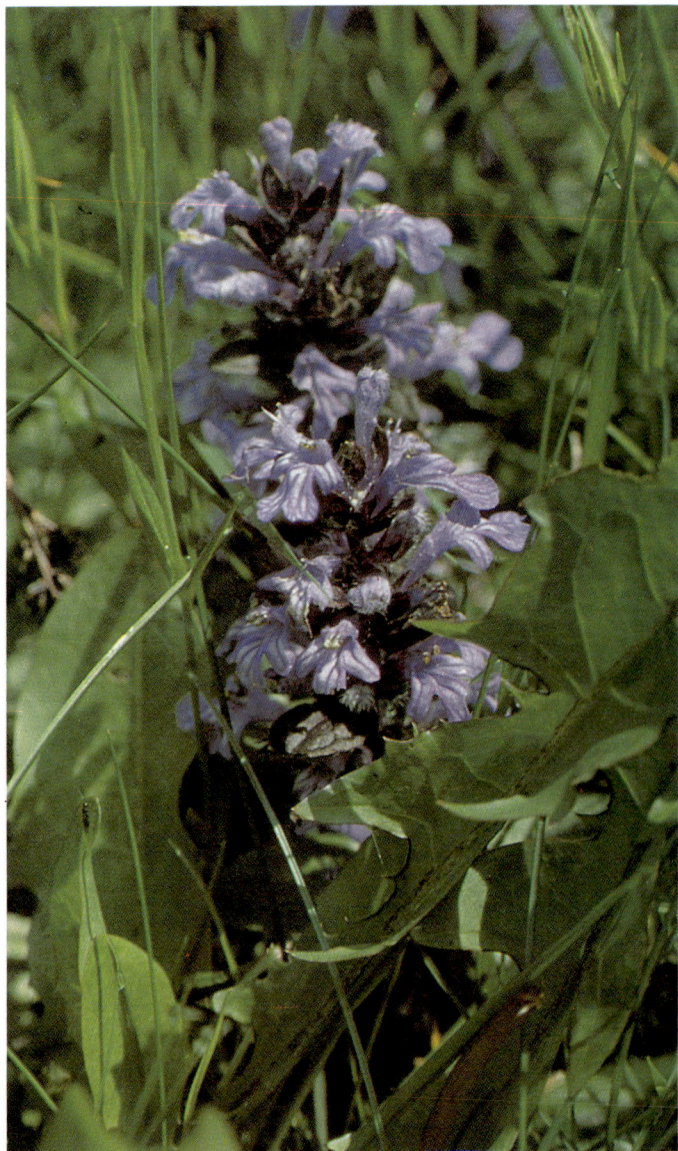

Carline thistle *(Carlina vulgaris)*

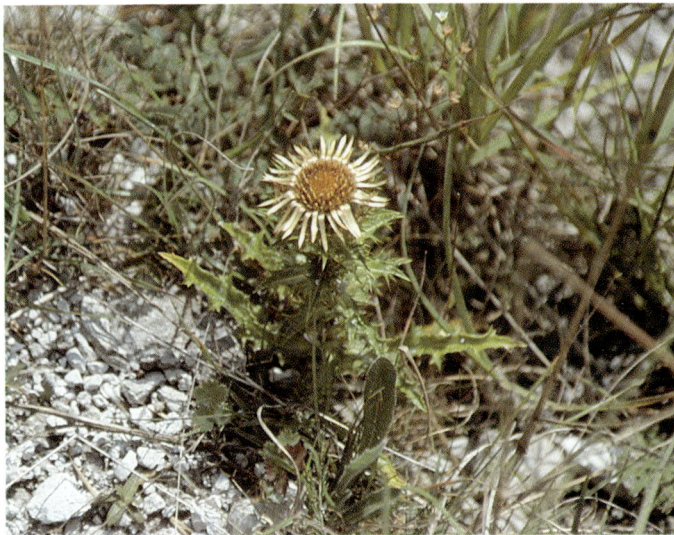

Coltsfoot *(Tussilago farfara)*

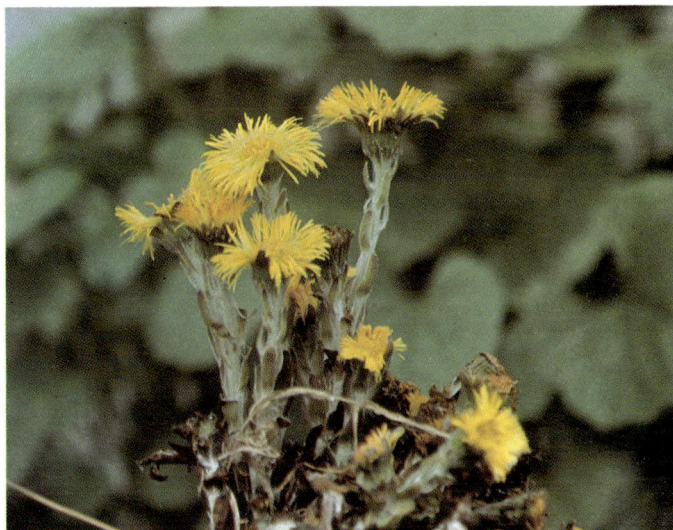

Evening primrose *(Oenothera biennis)*

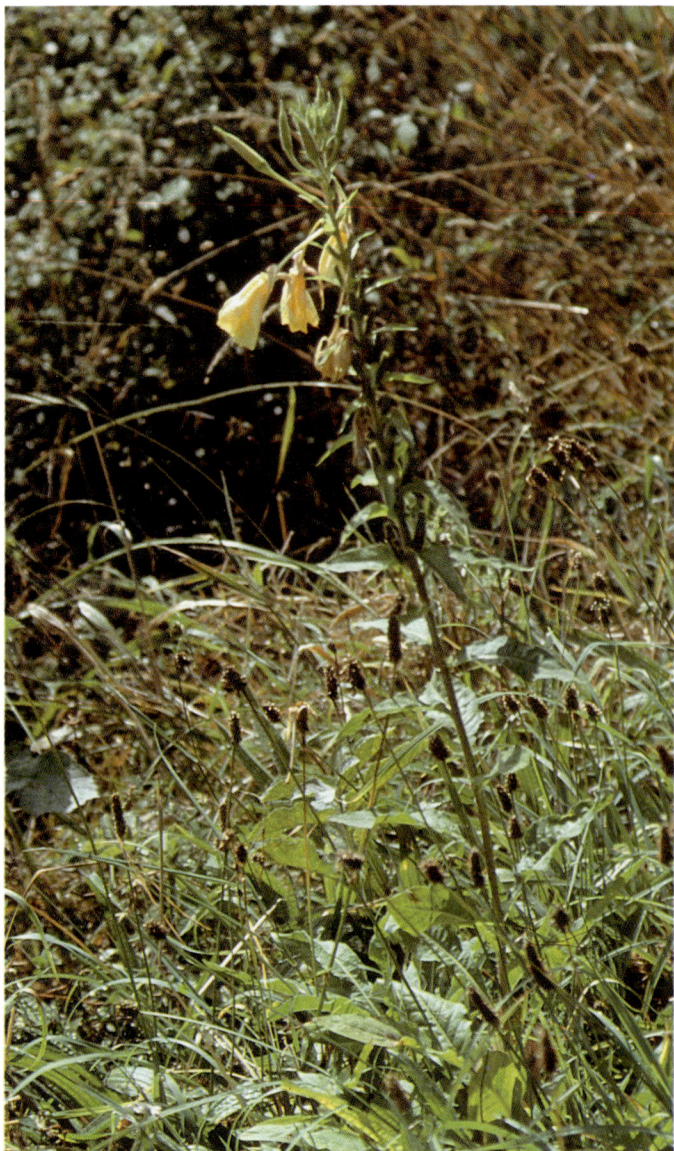

Fleabane *(Pulicaria dysenterica)*

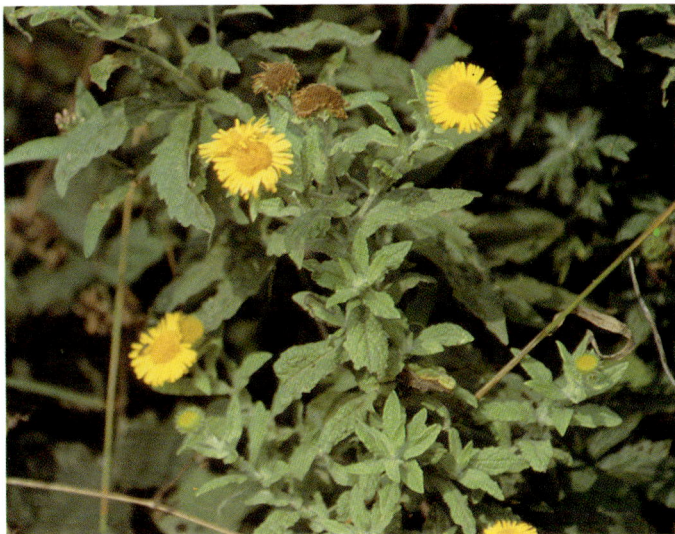

Knapweed *(Centaurea nigra)*

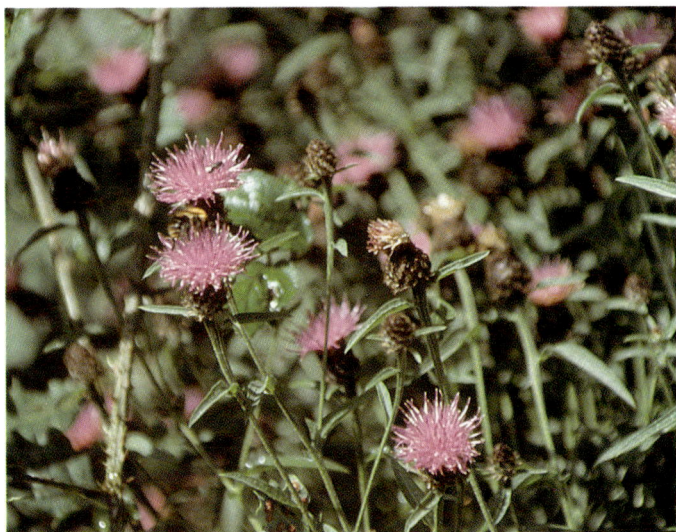

Common mallow *(Malva sylvestris)*

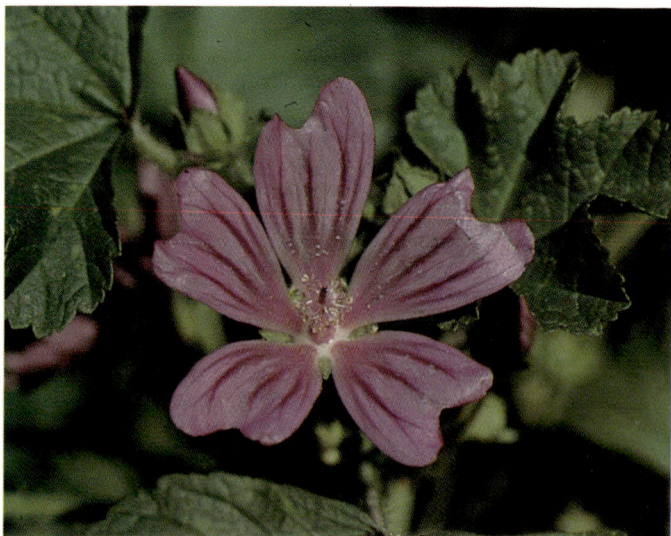

Old man's beard *(Clematis vitalba)*

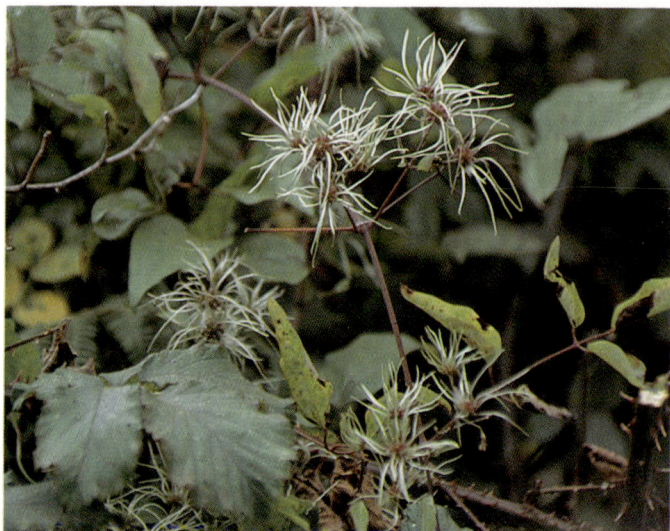

St John's wort *(Hypericum perforatum)*

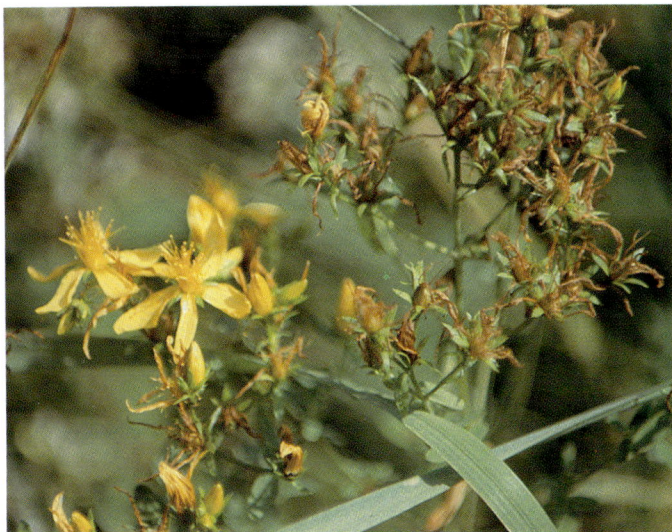

Pink and white valerian *(Centranthus ruber)*

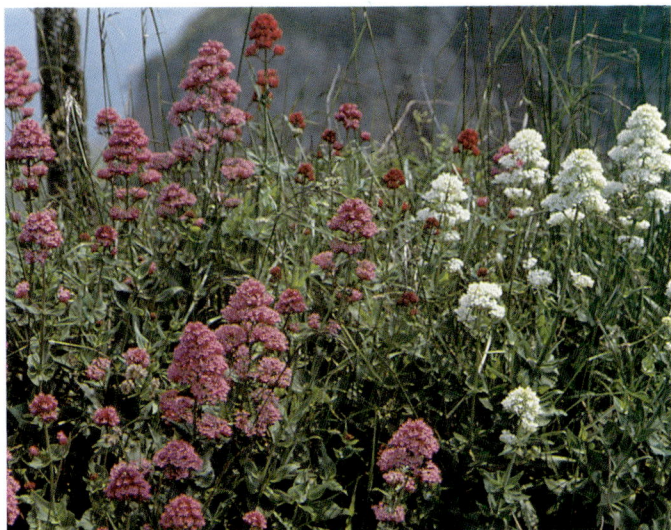

Yarrow *(Achillea millefolium)*

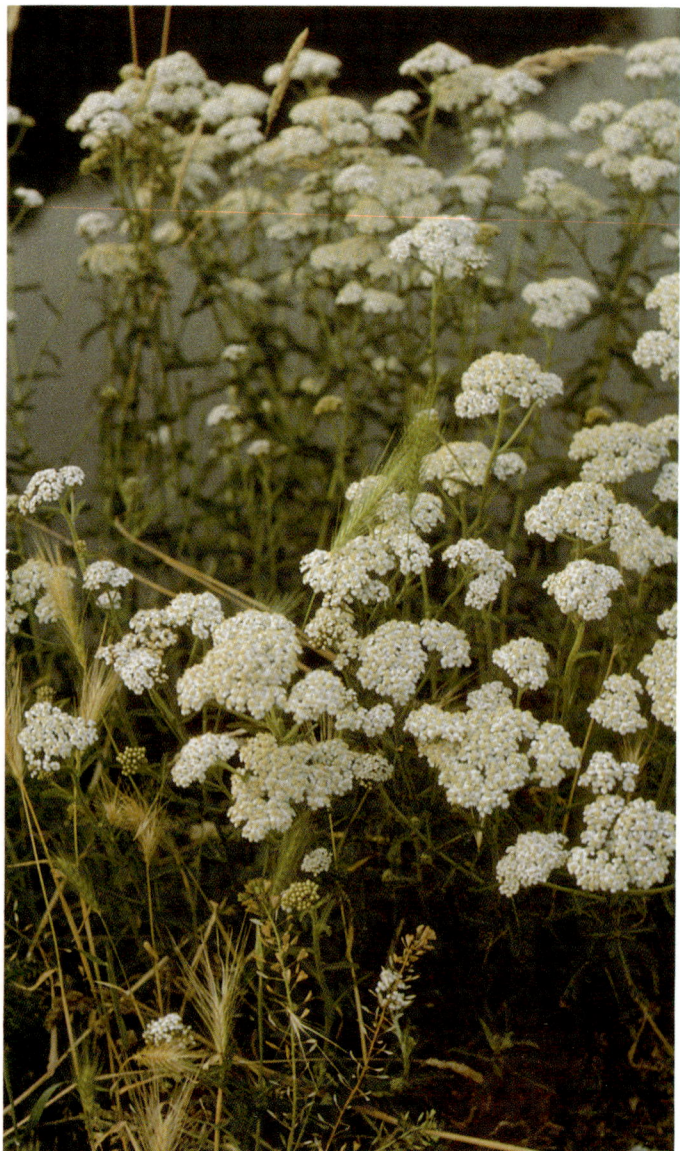

eye ointments, it was widely employed to poultice wounds and sprains, and American plants of the same family were adopted by the Indians to treat cancerous skin ulcers.

There are many ancient myths surrounding this simple weed of the daisy family. A particularly interesting one, which can have actual value if faith is strong enough, is the application of groundsel to cure toothache, as instructed by the Roman naturalist, Pliny the Elder. He said that if you uproot a plant of groundsel with your bare hands and touch the affected tooth with it, then replace the plant in the ground, it will begin to grow again, and as it grows so your tooth will cease aching. Possibly the tooth will have fallen out by then, anyway! Whatever the value of this remedy, there was sufficient faith in groundsel as a toothache cure to prompt Gerard to recommend it pressed in a little milk to sooth sore gums in young children.

Nowadays groundsel is more or less confined to a treatment for painful irregular periods in young girls. Homoeopathic doctors prescribe it for this purpose, and in France peasant girls are dosed with an infusion of groundsel to regularize periods and reduce menstrual pain.

The plant is used dried with the flowers intact; any seeding heads should be discarded. A handful of dried herb is steeped in 1 litre of boiling water, and a cupful should be taken 3 times a day. It has a less-than-pleasant taste which can be improved by adding a little honey.

Whether it had a beneficial effect on jaundice or cholera, for which it was prescribed in the sixteenth and seventeenth centuries, must be in some doubt, and there are few references to this aspect in herbals compiled after that time.

If this pernicious weed possesses even some of the powers that have been ascribed to it, then we should be pleased when the small deep-cut leaves appear in our flower beds. Somehow, though, I doubt we will be.

Heartsease
(Viola tricolor)
Family: VIOLACAEA

There are nearly two hundred members of this attractive family of plants. Some are found high up in the Himalayas and others on the lush lowland pastures of England's shire counties; consequently there is a considerable amount of folklore attached to them.

The flower looks rather like a human face and in some European countries a religious significance is given to it. It is sometimes known as the trinity herb because the petals are coloured white, blue and yellow. It's also called 'three faces in a wood', for the same reason.

Heartsease hybridizes freely and will appear in gardens almost as if

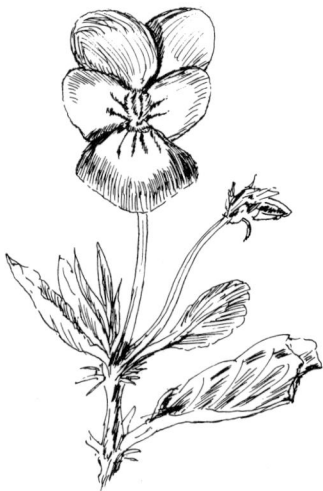

by magic, being a throwback to the original wild pansies known as heartsease crosses, and which actually form part of the lineage of garden cultivated varieties.

Pansies both wild and cultivated are blessed with healing properties, although when a plant is selectively bred for ornament its power for healing, other than the spirit, appears to be diminished.

As its name suggests, the herb was adopted for heart ailments, but its effect on any known heart disease is minimal, and under no circumstances should herbal preparations of any kind be taken for heart conditions without the full knowledge and agreement of your doctor.

However, a herbalist would prescribe heartsease for relieving minor pains and inflammation, as the plant contains derivatives of salicylic acid, the main ingredient of aspirin, and the smell of methyl salicylate (wintergreen) is quite noticeable when the plant is crushed or chewed.

The gentle action of heartsease is valuable in poultices for swollen joints and compresses, but in past times its main use was as a diuretic for ridding the body of excess fluid. It was one of the prime constituents in medicines for the dreaded condition of dropsy, itself a result of cardiac disorders. This is perhaps where heartsease derived its name.

Herbalists and laymen alike recommended wild pansy as a capital cleanser of blood at the changing of the seasons. A mild drink can be prepared by steeping 2 tablespoonfuls of dried whole flowering plant in 1 litre of cold water for 2 hours, then bringing gently to the boil. Remove from the heat and allow to brew for 10 minutes, drink immediately or bottle for later. Two or three cups per day is good for acne in adolescence, and this may well be one of the reasons why it was thought to cleanse the blood, but this effect could be due to its action as a diuretic.

Externally, applications of heartsease have proved invaluable, for under certain circumstances the active ingredients have a beneficial reaction on dry skin, especially eczema and psoriasis, by promoting healing.

There are many regional names for heartsease, from 'kiss-me-in-the-buttery' to 'banewort', so called because the Northumbrians considered there were few herbs better for bone healing than the shy heartsease.

When preparing wild pansies for storage, dry in an airing cupboard as quickly as possible. The root will continue growing after the plant has been pulled from the soil and washed, therefore if the upper flowering plant is dried separately there is less danger of mould forming and so rendering the herb useless. When thoroughly dry, crush gently over a clean white tissue, bottle in tightly closed glass containers and store in the dark. If brown glass containers are available this is even better.

Herb bennet

(Geum urbanum)
Family: ROSACEAE

Also known as wood avens, this small plant is considered a weed by most gardeners and as such is grubbed up from garden borders. Yet it has great herbal and medicinal value.

It's quite common, growing all over Europe, and found mainly in woodland margins, so it's easily obtainable and there is little reason to dry and store it. If you don't have free access to a garden or the countryside throughout the year it is possible to store this herb for future use by drying both root and leaves slowly in a warm shady place. The fresh root gives off a scent reminiscent of cloves, although this volatile ester vanishes as the root dries.

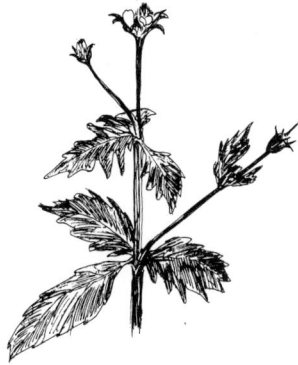

Herb bennet found favour during the Middle Ages, but it was well known to Greeks and Romans who used it for treating heart and liver ailments. Its greatest virtue is its safety, unlike some other herbal treatments for the heart such as foxglove which is a progressive poison and can build up in the body until it reaches dangerous levels.

However, the efficacy of herb bennet for heart ailments is unproven, and there are many reasons why people suffering from such a serious illness should not treat themselves with herbal preparations. This is a case where advice from a properly qualified medical practitioner should be sought.

There is a distinct possibility that the use of herb bennet for heart conditions came about because it was also prescribed for digestive ailments, with symptoms of heartburn and chronic wind.

The Romans held it in high regard for treating malaria, when it was used in much the same way as quinine for lowering temperature and preventing convulsions, and also for relieving diarrhoea and its attendant dehydration. They prepared the herb in wine by soaking 40g of crushed root in 1 litre of wine for 6 days in a tightly stoppered bottle. Then it was strained and taken 1 glassful 3 times a day.

As a mild tonic for a sensitive stomach, add 30g of fresh ground root to 1 litre of boiling water. Steep for 10 minutes and drink a cupful 3 times a day until the condition abates.

An infusion of fresh root is also handy as an antiseptic for minor wounds and grazes, and was thought to be a suitable external treatment for spots and non-allergic skin conditions.

The plant itself is quite attractive, with leaves and flowers similar in shape to wild strawberry. The yellow flowers are borne singly at the tips of the stalk and open during May and June. It can be grown easily from seed gathered in July, when the capsule is ripe, to ensure an uncontaminated supply of the root.

Gardeners may be less than enthusiastic about this lowly plant, but it once occupied an honoured place in medicine and was said to have stronger active properties if it grew in hilly areas with clean air.

Hollyhock

(Althaea rosea)
Family: MALVACEAE

The tall flowering spikes of hollyhocks are typical of the English country garden. The plant is a member of the mallow family, and some of the properties of that family are attributed to it, such as calming the digestive system. The colour of a flower sometimes appears to have some connection with its value medicinally; in this case the dark purple petals containing anthocyanin pigment.

In the past, hollyhock flowers have been gathered as a constituent in medicines to ease bronchitis symptoms, and one of the benefits of the infused flowers is that they lend a pleasing burgundy colour to a herbal brew. These flower pigments found favour with the wine trade in past years for enriching the colour of wine.

Biennial or perennial, the first year's growth is limited to establishing a basal rosette of leaves whereon the second year's flower spike is formed. In favourable conditions the plant can grow to over 2m.

It is thought that hollyhocks are one of the oldest garden cultivars. They are not a native of England, but are seemingly numbered among those plants the Romans introduced into this country during their long occupation. There is little doubt that Romano-British settlers established the plant for its

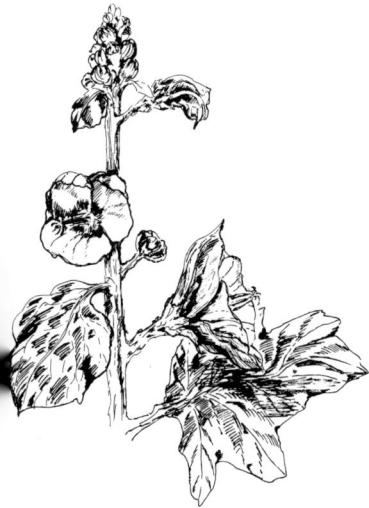

there is little or nothing in the plant's active constituents to justify this.

Honeysuckle

(Lonicera periclymenum)
Family: CAPRIFOLIACEAE

In 1837 the French sage Roques observed that it was a good thing for people recovering from an illness to be able to go out into the countryside to some quiet balmy spot and breathe in fresh air scented with the perfume of honeysuckle – in fact he called it woodbine, the common country name for this plant.

For centuries poets have sung the praises of its beauty and its perfume. In Shakespeare's *A Midsummer Night's Dream*, Queen Titania murmurs to Nick Bottom, the weaver, who is bewitched, 'Sleep thou, and I will wind thee in my arms. So doth woodbine the sweet honeysuckle gently entwist.' Shakespeare was obviously familiar with this plant, for at that time the main plant was called woodbine, the sweetly perfumed flowers being the honeysuckle.

It must have been very common in the sixteenth century, for England was heavily wooded then, and as its name suggests, woodbine grows in woodlands, twisting itself around hazel and hardwood saplings in a green and gold cascade. However, the peasant herbalists of Shakespeare's England were generally more concerned with

decorative as well as its medicinal properties.

It grows naturally in the Middle East and is much prized by Bedouin tribes, being administered to prevent miscarriage, although this action has never been proven. For many years, however, it was used for uterine infections, vaginitis and threatened miscarriage.

Mucilage contained in the leaves can be prepared in the same way as mallow for soothing the digestion after upsets, and both leaves and flowers can be employed in the preparation of a lotion to ease dry itching skin and for treating sunburn, providing the skin is unbroken. This lotion will soothe an inflamed area.

There are records of the leaves and flowers of hollyhocks being used as a worm treatment, but

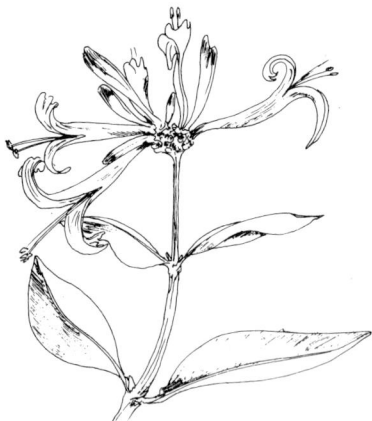

perties are better supplied by modern drugs and antibiotics. Bronchitis sufferers would be unwise to attempt to treat themselves with honeysuckle these days.

There is no doubt that had the Victorians had access to modern antibiotics then that other scourge of rich and poor alike, pneumonia, would not have wreaked such havoc.

Hops
(Humulus lupulus)
Family: CANNABACEAE

honeysuckle's potential as a medicine than with its beauty.

The medicinal properties of the plant are in fact more than you might imagine. The leaves and flower buds are rich in salicylic acid, the active ingredient in aspirin. An infusion of honeysuckle leaves was used to relieve the symptoms of influenza, reducing temperature and easing the accompanying headache.

For centuries bronchitis was know as the English disease, caused by the climate and poor living conditions of most of the population. In consequence, recourse to honeysuckle was common to relieve the coughing spasms that afflicted the poor, undernourished children of working people in field and foundry. Another ingredient found in the leaves is a natural antibiotic useful in helping intestinal ailments.

Now most of its healing pro-

Being the source of the main flavouring agent in beer, this scrambling vine-like plant has become an established part of the culture of Western society. The cone-like fruiting bodies produce the aromatic resin used in beers to give a bitter taste and improve keeping qualities.

It is common in the countryside, having escaped from cultivation, but has a chequered history. It was known as a medicinal ingredient in a type of ale drunk by the Jews in Babylon to protect themselves against leprosy, and the Romans cultivated it for the young growing tips which they ate as vegetables — a practice which still exists.

The use of hops in beer appears to have begun in England in the ninth or tenth centuries, but later the court of Henry VIII was so much against their use that they were banned as an ingredient in

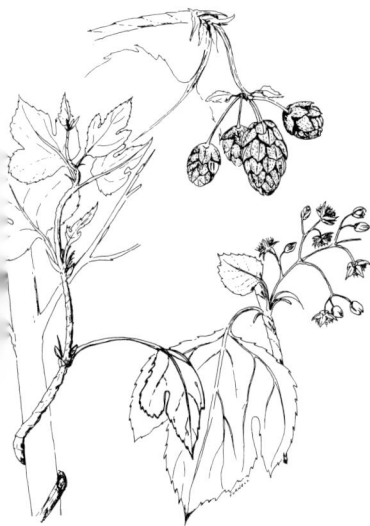

cultivation, they were prescribed as a sedative, and hop pillows are an old country remedy for insomnia. Lupulin, a bitter yellow extract of hops, is known for its sedative qualities and especially for its depressant action on men's sexual activity. It appears that this compound has the opposite effect on women, which is perhaps why beer drinking by both sexes is less than compatible!

Horse chestnut
(Aesculus hippocastanum)
Family: HIPPOCASTANACEAE

In spring the spire-like pink or white nectar-rich flowers of horse chestnuts attract the first questing bumblebees, yet this glorious tree is not a native of northern Europe; it comes originally from the Indian sub-continent. Its medicinal qualities, rather than its beauty, led to the planting of so many avenues of horse chestnuts.

It has certain properties found most particularly in the nut in early autumn. The bitter taste left on your hands after handling split and damaged conker skins comes from a toxin known as aesculin or aescine. This compound is a recognized poison and there have been instances, happily quite rare, when it has caused illness in young children who have ignored the bitter taste and eaten the skin together with some of the nut inside. The flesh of the nut can be made edible, but only after a long

beer, and this ban remained in force until the reign of Edward VI.

It has been known for hundreds of years that the resin in hops preserves beer for a considerable period of time, but the diarist John Evelyn in the seventeenth century believed that hops as a preservative would be extremely bad for the user. Yet the plant was employed medicinally to ease the symptoms of sexually transmitted diseases such as gonorrhoea – perhaps partly because it is an aphrodisiac and lessened sexual desire! It was also recommended for yellow jaundice, as a worm treatment for intestinal parasites, and to relieve itching and dry scabby skin.

In the United States, where hops are also found as escapees from

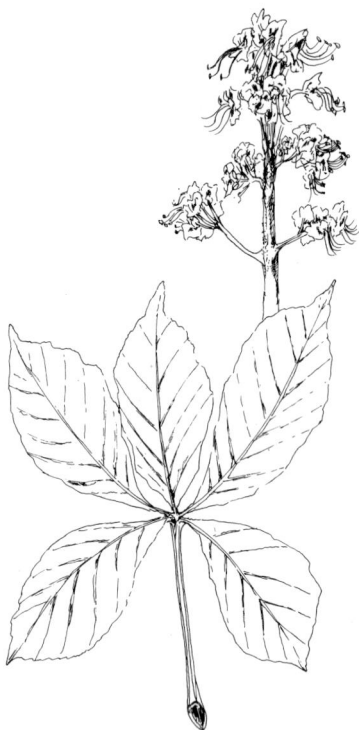

and laborious process.

North American Indians are experts at utilizing products of the forest. They use horse chestnut as a food, rendering the poison harmless by first cooking and washing the floury paste made from the nuts in a wicker basket under running water. When the flour is dried it's said to be palatable; there is also a method of treating cooked and ground horse chestnut flour with alcohol to remove the aesculin.

During the Second World War the inhabitants of occupied countries roasted and ground the nuts to make a coffee substitute; although bitter it was just about bearable. The flesh of the nut is starchy and ferments readily to form a fiery spirit which can be distilled, but this is no longer done. Moreover, the tree buds have been used to flavour drinks and there are records of their being substituted for hops in brewing beer.

However, horse chestnut has many other uses. Indian herbalists recommended extract of horse chestnut for treating that most disabling of bodily conditions, haemorrhoids, and the related symptoms of swollen and varicose veins. Extract of horse chestnut is not recommended in home-made herbal preparations, as misuse could be dangerous. Nevertheless, prescribed by a qualified practitioner in the right proportions it has helped to relieve distress caused by painful and bleeding piles, and it's likely that one very famous sufferer from this complaint, Napoleon Bonaparte, had recourse to such a remedy.

The name 'horse chestnut' derives from the horseshoe-shaped scar left on the twig after the leaf has fallen in autumn. In Turkey, horse chestnut was administered to restore the staying power of broken-winded horses.

In France the dried ground nuts were adopted as a snuff to promote sneezing, which was considered a health-restoring reflex, and French washerwomen used the saponin content of horse chestnut as a soap to launder clothes. When treated in this way they resisted storage mould and insect infestation. This particular property and the bitter taste led to its utilization as a size for treating wooden furniture where the surface of the timber was open to attack from furniture beetles.

There have been many cases in history when starvation was staved off by exploiting the horse chestnuts as food, and the muscular strain and illnesses brought on by hard work could be lessened with an extract of nuts or even bark from young twigs.

Faith in this tree was so strong that peasants often carried horse chestnuts in their pocket as a remedy for rheumatism. The active ingredients were thought to be so powerful that as they dried this power would pass into the body, and the nuts were removed only when they were completely dry and hard as stone. Faith and autosuggestion in simple minds can sometimes affect the most miraculous cures.

Horseradish

(Armoracia rusticana)
Family: CRUCIFERAE

The roast beef of old England added greatly to our ancestors' digestive ailments, and it was for this reason, plus the fact that a large carcass took a long time to consume and without the benefit of refrigeration would quickly deteriorate, that the traditional method of preserving beef was to salt it. This was at best a difficult art, and at worst a licence to poison the consumers.

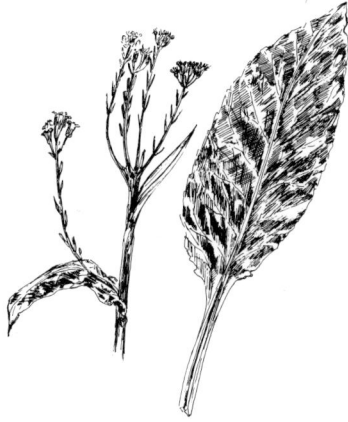

The least palatable beef from old cows and draft oxen usually went into salting for consumption by the Navy, so it's something of a miracle that the British won any sea battles at all. Presumably the food supplied to the enemy was even worse.

At home the autumnal kill of animals for smoking and salting led to a surfeit of protein for an undernourished population, but they could eat only so much at a sitting. After a while the meat would begin to go off, and flavouring was needed to improve smell and taste. The flavours available then would be familiar to us now, especially eastern herbs and spices, which were a main feature of cooking and helped to make rancid food edible.

It was not until the seventeenth century that horseradish was introduced to provide what has now become a traditional flavouring to complement roast beef. The root of horseradish is the part used by cooks and herbalists alike, as the large fleshy green leaves are rather too pungent to eat, although the plant comes from the same group as cabbage.

In some places horseradish plants have colonized a complete area after escaping the cultivated confines of a herb garden, often becoming a common weed when growing on rich soil.

Many properties have been ascribed to the root, and although one of these is that it stimulates secretion of digestive juices when used in small quantities, large amounts can cause stomach upsets, for the mustard oil which is freely liberated when the root is chopped or grated can inflame the sensitive lining of the gut.

For many years it was prescribed to stimulate circulation and because of this horseradish was, and still is, used in herbal preparations to reduce cold or flu symptoms.

Grated root can be made into a cough syrup for bronchial catarrh. (You may prefer to grate the root out of doors, as it is irritant to the eyes, nose and throat.) Scrape some fresh root into a clean bowl and cover with sugar; turn frequently for a day until there is a layer of syrup at the bottom of the bowl.

This should be drained off into a clean bottle and labelled clearly. Take 3 times a day, 1 tablespoon at a time.

Its benefits are said to come from the root's ability to increase the blood flow to tissues and remove waste products from the body. Together with its antiseptic properties, this has caused it to be widely used in Europe for treating boils.

The root is sliced and placed on the swelling and renewed every hour with fresh applications, but be careful: horseradish juice can irritate sensitive skins and cause blistering, particularly if slices of root are put on sore joints as a relief for rheumatism.

Horsetail
(Equisetum arvense)
Family: EQUISETACEAE

Field horsetail has a multitude of names, among them 'pewterwort', for it was the plant's usefulness in cleaning pewter that caused it to be encouraged in many a medieval garden.

The stems of horsetail are unusual in that the tissue is supported by a network of crystals of silica. Indeed, this is a plant with a skeleton, and a history almost as long as life itself. In the coal measures and the shales of four hundred million years ago there are clear traces of a plant so similar to horsetail as to be indistinguish-

family, it reproduces by means of spores; these spring from a fruiting body during April which dies away before the bottle-brush leafy stems develop.

These stems and their silica crystals were a constituent of pewter polish and many metal polishes used during the Middle Ages. In fact, you can't do much better today for soft metal than to use horsetail. When the leaves and stems are dried and burned the ash is found to contain a great deal of silica, approximately 80% by weight. This powdered ash, mixed with water, puts a shine on silver like the one it had when it left the silversmith.

To use horsetail simply as a silver polish would cause herbalists of bygone days to turn in their graves. From the time of the Romans and Greeks onwards there is a wealth of information about this useful plant.

The Romans especially used fresh tender tips of young horsetail in a tonic salad. Analysis has shown that apart from the bitter flavour which makes the plant so unpalatable to animals – an excellent method of self-preservation – the plant contains other minerals than silica in an easily assimilated form.

A lotion of horsetail was employed to stop bleeding, but it was as a medicine for bronchial infections that the early English herbalists included it in their pharmacy. They soaked the stems in 1 litre of water for 3 hours, then boiled them

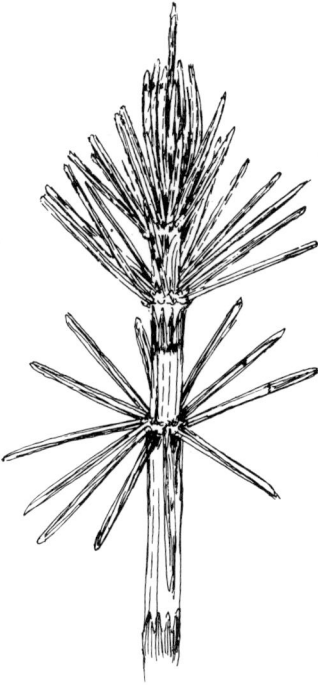

able from the one that grows today, were it not for one important detail. The coal measure plants were forty-odd feet high, with the dimensions and appearance of pine trees. They had a vast far-seeking root system that reclaimed marshland and provided a habitat for dragonflies with a wingspan almost a metre across.

Modern-day horsetail is less spectacular in scale, but is still valued for its medicinal qualities by herbalists and homoeopathic practitioners.

It is a rather strange plant in that, like members of the fern

for 20 minutes. The brew was then left to cool before straining. Several cups of this potion were to be taken during the day, and it was recommended for a persistent cough. Naturally, anyone suffering from a persistent cough today would be advised to visit their doctor rather than treat themselves, but in the past there was no recourse to our modern miracle drugs.

Another valuable property of this plant was to replace minerals lacking in some diets. The same decoction as for coughs was prescribed in this case, with 3 cups to be taken per day. It was supposed to prevent flaking and splitting fingernails.

Horsetail seems to have been classed as a cure-all with an impressive, if unlikely, list of potent cures to its credit, from cut sinews to gastric ulcers. Yet it was for rheumatism, gout and similar illnesses that it was most widely advocated, and it is referred to in herbals as a remedy for gallstones and gravel. (Nowadays it is widely used by herbalists for many diseases of the kidneys and bladder.)

As a concentrate, that is to say, the liquid prepared as above but with from 50g to 100g of stems to $\frac{1}{2}$ litre of water, it speeded healing, prevented dry and flaking skin from cracking, healed ulcers, and, if sniffed up the nose, was supposed to stop nosebleeds immediately.

Records concerning horsetail have been found in many countries, which must surely indicate that there is some real value in the plant for the purposes of herbal remedies. However, there could also be an element of self-preservation here, promoted by past herbalists who were troubled by rampant horsetail growth in their herb gardens. How much better it would be to convince their clients that it was valuable as a medicine rather than spend hours of back-breaking toil trying to eradicate the pest!

Hyssop
(Hyssopus officinalis)
Family: LABIATAE

Hyssop is the plant that the Roman soldier is supposed to have used to hold up the sponge soaked in vinegar to Jesus on the Cross.

It was a well known culinary herb in Britain, originating in the Middle East and the drier areas of the Mediterranean. Classed as a shrub, it is actually a member of the same family as mint, sage and balm, and is a tough, low-growing, rather woody plant that does well in sunny gardens.

The flowers are of the typical labiate form, very attractive, and blue or pink. The foliage is smoky-green and when crushed in the hand exudes a pleasant odour echoed by the scent of the flowers. It is often grown as an ornamental plant, and although severe frosts may affect it, will usually continue

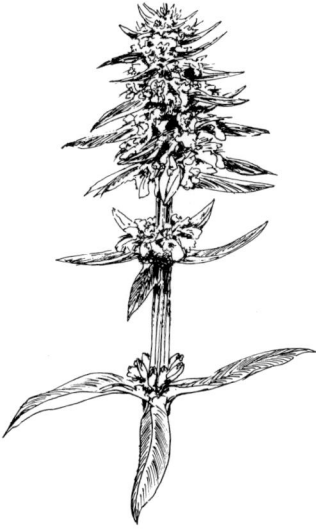

to grow vigorously for a number of years.

Where grown for medicinal purposes it will normally be dug up and removed every four years and replaced with seedlings.

The flavour is rather acrid, and although it was very popular in cooking and for preserving in the Middle Ages, it is less popular nowadays. The advent of refrigeration has meant that meat doesn't go off so easily, and this is what the strong aromatic taste of hyssop was intended to disguise.

Although its culinary popularity is in decline, it is still used by herbalists for bronchitis, asthma and pleurisy, and in the company of other herbs of the same family is helpful in reducing cold symptoms.

It is also an expectorant, and the Greeks, masters of herbal treatment in the early days of written history, advised that it should be boiled in water and honey and given to relieve tightness of the chest. Gerard mentions a recipe where figs and honey boiled in water with hyssop could be taken to ease persistent coughs.

As well as the leaves and flowers being employed in cough and cold remedies, dried powdered root was also used to ease liver and spleen infections and for jaundice. Although these illnesses are far too serious to treat yourself without properly qualified medical advice, in the days before national health care systems, hyssop root was invaluable.

The root contains several bitter glycosides considered helpful for gout sufferers, and there is some basis for this belief in the fact that these glycosides are somewhat diuretic in action and may also be administered to reduce temperature in certain conditions.

There can be some side-effects, and if hyssop root is taken in large doses, sickness and diarrhoea may result. It is a stimulant that will irritate the stomach, and in some rare cases cause violent purging; hence perhaps the passage in the Bible where David says 'Purge me with hyssop,' although nowadays it is believed that a species of spurge may have been intended.

Iris

*(Iris foetidissima, Iris
pseudacorus)*

Family: IRIDACEAE

USA: yellow flag (*pseudacorus*)

Members of the iris family have
been symbols of royalty since rul-
ing families became a feature of
civilization in Europe and the
Middle East. Iris flowers are depicted in paintings on tomb walls in
the Valley of the Kings, and this
symbolic flower is used as the
decoration on the Sphinx's brow.

The flowers are thought to have
been used as a model for the fleur
de lis or fleur de luce of the French
kings, and the design of three
feathers on the arms of the Prince
of Wales is very close to the configuration of a common flag iris.

The large showy flowers thrive
where there is an ample supply of
water and mud, and bloom well in
the damp steamy atmosphere of the
Nile delta. The Greeks took iris to
their hearts, for it is such a fine
flower and they thought its sharp
symbolic sword-shaped leaves
must link it with the gods. The
flowers were popular as votive
offerings at the altar of many gods
and goddesses, especially the goddess of the rainbow and messenger
of gods, Iris.

Iris seeds are contained in a pod
at the top of a tall stem. When ripe,
this pod splits to reveal bright-red
bead-like seeds which can be
roasted to provide a reasonable
substitute for coffee.

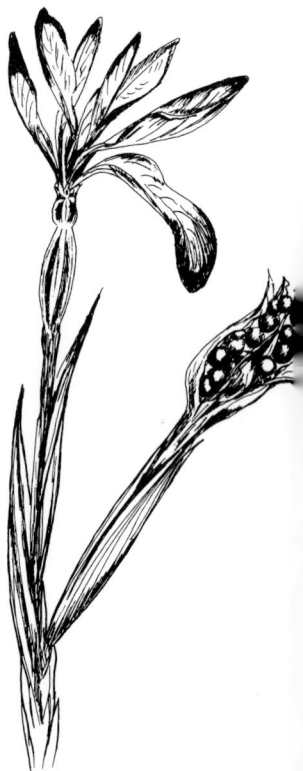

Sadly, the wild iris most widely
known in Britain is stinking iris. Its
name derives from the smell
emanating from the juice of the cut
leaves, which some people find
repulsive, whilst others find it
quite acceptable.

In the Middle Ages the smell was
considered similar to roast beef – in
fact, it was known as 'the roast beef
plant'. This gives us some insight
into those days when beef was
hung for long periods of time prior

to eating. It's likely that joints of meat were very high before our ancestors consumed them, which may account, in part, for the high death rate and explain why so many remedies found in ancient herbals are for relief of gastric upsets and diarrhoea. Culpeper states in his herbal that the root of iris is good for cleansing the body of 'fluxes', a sixteenth- and seventeenth-century term for diarrhoea.

The old English name of 'spurge-wort' also gives an insight into the uses for which iris root was employed. The strong-smelling bitter root is a powerful purgative and can cause severe irritation of the gut.

Many medicines were administered to procure abortions, and when used as a pessary or taken as a draught iris root and honey was considered convenient because of this purging property. Many women suffered greatly and even then failed to achieve the desired result. Some, debilitated by poverty and weakened by the effects of iris root, died from resulting loss of blood and secondary infection. This was one of the unfortunate aspects of medicinal misuse of plant remedies, and many so-called apothecaries were heartless charlatans preying on the ignorant.

Nevertheless, iris had a role to play, in fact it still has, for powdered root of florentine iris (*Iris florentina*), better known as orris plant, forms the basis of most violet-scented perfumes.

The root is unusual in that it has to be dried before it will release its aroma, and in Florence it used to be chewed to dispel bad breath and calm the stomach – though its calming effects must be called into doubt because of its purgative qualities.

Ivy, common
(Hedera helix)
Family: ARALIACEAE

In the distant past, the Druids and their precursors revered several plants which they believed to possess great spiritual powers. One of the most potent was ivy, and it would appear that all over northern Europe this tough scrambling climber was looked upon with favour, perhaps because in a deep, cold winter ivy is one of the few plants to retain fresh green leaves; even its flowers bloom until very late in the year and can be found open to any passing insect even in November.

The rather insignificant yellow-green flowers are sweetly scented and rich in nectar and were once gathered as an ingredient for cough remedies.

In Roman times the God Bacchus was depicted wearing a wreath of ivy on his head, and a crown of ivy was considered to be a good cure for drunkenness. This may have been the reason why in some areas in the Middle Ages ivy stems were gathered to make goblets.

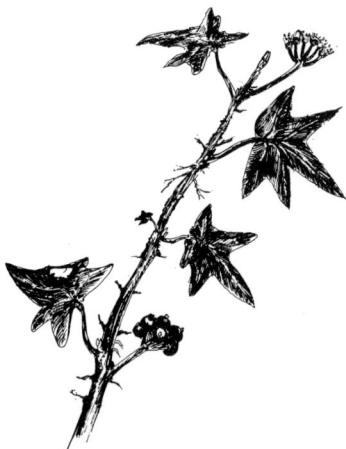

During the great plagues, an infusion of ivy berries in wine was recommended as a remedy for this dread disease. This probably added to the suffering of plague victims and hastened their end, for the berries are a powerful purgative, but in those days it was thought that remedies which caused sneezing or vomiting were of benefit in ridding the body of so-called ill humours.

Medicinally speaking, ivy is fraught with danger, especially the berries. It should never be taken internally, for it contains several toxic substances and there is some evidence to suggest that it can cause anaemia through the destruction of red corpuscles. It is best to avoid using the berries even externally, as they are toxic and irritant.

Despite the existence of these dangers, there are many old re-medies using the leaves for sore throats, mouth ulcers and whooping cough which advocate an infusion of ivy leaves to be taken internally. Externally, the leaves can be used to treat rheumatic conditions, both as a cold compress, where chopped leaves are applied to the affected area, or as a hot poultice. For the latter, mix a handful of chopped leaves with a handful of bran moistened with boiling water, fold in a cloth and apply as hot as can be borne to the affected place. This same poultice is said to be excellent for treating boils and abcesses.

Juniper
(Juniperus communis)
Family: CUPRESSACEAE

USA: hack matack, juniper, horse savin

Although commonly grown in gardens all over the northern hemisphere, juniper is actually a native of rocky countryside, preferring the high stark terrain of Europe, northern Asia and north America.

It has a long, well-documented history, for juniper fronds were burned in the streets of Athens on Hippocrates' instructions in an attempt to keep the plague at bay, and indeed the same means of disinfection was employed by Parisians in the 1870 smallpox epidemic, when fronds were burned in hospitals.

It is likely that the tree Hippo-

flavouring to gin, the social scourge of the poor in the eighteenth century. There were more deaths attributed to the effects of this pernicious spirit than to the agency of infectious disease. Yet an extract of juniper berry has great therapeutic qualities as an internal medicine.

Juniper berries are made into an infusion with 40g of berries to 1 litre of boiling water. Soak for 10 minutes and strain. This was once used as a remedy for renal colic, dyspepsia, disorders of the prostrate gland and cystitis, but modern herbalists avoid prescribing it for any kidney disorder or for pregnant women.

The same infusion can also be used as an external lotion for dry irritated skins, although the usual warnings about skin sensitivity should be borne in mind and the mixture patch-tested on a small area of skin before application.

It is also recommended for treating rheumatism and gout, although usually externally, with branches and berries used to make a compress. One recipe suggests 250g of fronds and branch to 2 litres of boiling water. Boil for 2 hours and then apply to the affected area as a compress, as hot as comfortable. This brew has quite a marked antiseptic property and has been used in cases of varicose ulcers as a cleansing wash.

Oil of juniper is available from chemists and herbalists to treat rheumatism, and as already mentioned, vapour of juniper is a well-

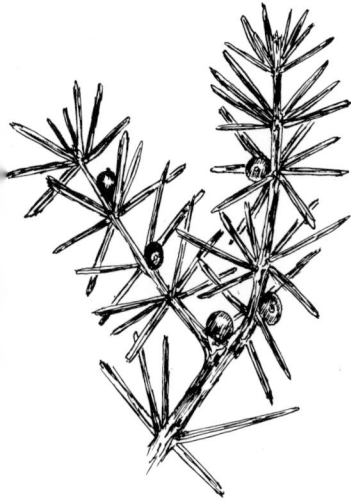

crates was familiar with was the Syrian juniper (*Juniperus drupaceae*). Records show that Hannibal ordered a temple to be built with a juniper-wood roof, and there are many Greek historical documents advocating juniper wood for building because it is extremely resistant to rot.

Common juniper wood could not have fulfilled the role of roof support for the Temple of Diana, for although it possesses rot-resisting qualities similar to its Syrian cousin, it rarely grows more than 4m tall and the unbranched trunk is often no more than 2m in height.

Being diminutive in size does not prevent the common juniper from being a giant as far as history and medicine are concerned. The black fleshy fruits were added as a

known fumigant. If branches are burned in a sickroom the vapours can have a soothing quality. Check with your medical practitioner, however, before attempting this.

Kidney vetch
(Anthyllis vulneraria)
Family: LEGUMINOSAE

Commonly found on chalk soils, providing they have not been fertilized, this ground cover plant comes from a family well-known for its ability to fix nitrogen from the air into the soil, so making it available to other plants.

Kidney vetch actually colonizes the ground and is capable of growing on bare chalk where no other plants can get a toe-hold.

Medicinally it has been explored very little, perhaps because of its habit of growing in isolation and in hostile ground conditions which man and animals avoid.

In the past shepherds used the plant, which is also known as 'ladies' fingers' because the flowers look like a hand in a woollen glove. They used it to salve cuts on sheep's udders caused by brambles, and also to treat sore teats.

The flowers appear at the height of June and should be dried in the sun and taken as a tea to soothe mouth ulcers. They can also be applied to treat cuts and bruises. The seeds may be sown in the same manner as mustard and cress and added to salads, for they are rich in minerals and vitamins.

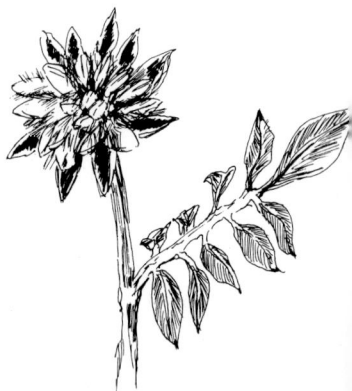

Please don't gather wild kidney vetch, for it is the sole larval food of several rare and endangered species of butterfly, particularly the small blue. The seeds are freely available from many nurseries and seedsmen.

Knapweed
(Centaurea nigra)
Family: COMPOSITAE

A cheerful attractive plant of chalk downland and waste places, knapweed belongs to the same family as thistles; indeed the flowerheads are very similar to thistle, but without the prickles. It is a favourite with butterflies, which will home in on it from a great distance, and if you plant it in a herb garden there will be plenty of colour from insect visitors.

Knapweed has been used to stay bleeding, and many older herbals state that a decoction of knapweed will stop vaginal haemorrhage and also bleeding piles, but there are considerable dangers in treating such symptoms without knowledge of the underlying cause.

In fifteenth and sixteenth century herbals there is reference to the application of knapweed in treating cancers, but again there is much danger in misinterpretation of the original meaning, for there are instances in these old herbals when 'cancers' and 'tumours' were words used to describe non-malignant ailments such as boils or abcesses. Anyone applying these flowers to treat malignant skin conditions will have no success and could actually delay modern treatment, which might effect a cure if caught in the early stages.

The root is accredited with the power to relieve dropsy, as it contains a mild diuretic, and the seeds and root in combination are thought to have tonic properties. Young fresh flowerheads can be eaten in salads and make a pleasant addition to a natural salad in summer time. A yellow-green dye can be extracted from the flowerheads by boiling with an alum mordant.

Culpeper recommended tea made by boiling 28g of grated root in 1 litre of water for 20 minutes, as a treatment for catarrh. It should be taken a tablespoonful at a time.

The reputation of the flower, root and leaf of knapweed to stay bleeding is worthy of further investigation, and an ointment can be made by digesting the flowers and leaves in a little wax. The powdered root can also be treated in this way and is said to be excellent for cuts and bruises.

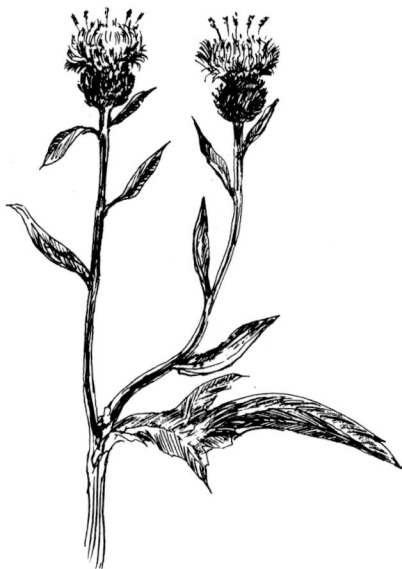

Both flowers and leaf can also be prepared for the relief of stomach upsets caused by overeating. Boil a handful of fresh plant in $\frac{1}{2}$ litre of water. Allow to cool, and strain. Take a wineglass at a time. This is also effective as a gargle for sore throats.

There are a number of closely related species of knapweed, including common large knapweed (*Centaurea scabiosa*) and knapwort (*Centaurea jacea*). They all seem to share similar properties.

Knotgrass

(Polygonum aviculare)
Family: POLYGONACEAE

This is not in fact a grass, neither is it knotted, and although exceedingly common in many habitats it has become one of the most neglected of all herbal cures.

It is so small and insignificant in appearance that it's hardly surprising it has fallen from favour, but it was much appreciated in the past, and the usual rule of thumb which suggests that the properties of any given plant are in proportion to its number of common names certainly applies here, for as well as being known as 'coral necklace' because of the tufts of coral-pink flowers which grow from the axis of each leaf joint, it is also called 'knotweed', 'irongrass', 'sparrow tongue' and 'doorweed', to name just a few. There are at least five more names.

It is a born survivor and common in sub-species throughout the world. In China, the home of herbal medicine today, there is a method of extracting a blue dye from dried knotgrass leaves by boiling them with alum.

Medicinally, it yields a fairly high level of tannin, which makes it good for treating diarrhoea and digestive tract infections. It is also said to be an excellent, if somewhat variable, remedy for acute symptoms of cystitis. The stems are rich in minerals, especially silica, in a readily assimilated form, and they have been recommended in the past for alleviating tuberculosis.

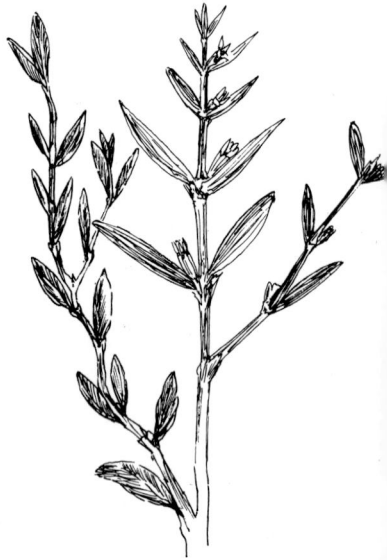

The stems, which can reach a length of 1m, are applied as an external poultice. They should be washed clean, for they are low-growing and frequently splashed with soil and foreign matter. The washed stems are boiled in a little water for 10 minutes until they are pulpy. This pulp can be applied to sores that are slow to heal and will also arrest bleeding.

Leek

(Allium porrum)
Family: LILIACEAE

It seems that attitudes towards leeks depend upon where in the world you live. In the south and south-west of England leeks are regarded merely as vegetables, a flavouring and an addition to winter stews.

However, in the part of England north of the Wash there is a hint of reverence in the attitude of the average man in the street to this tall and stately member of the onion clan. Go even further north, and the leek is king among vegetables, prized and cossetted and grown to massive proportions. These aristocratic plants are destined not only to fill the bellies of the Black Countrymen and their families; they are grown to be shown on benches at garden produce shows.

How and why the leek became such a popular vegetable is hard to understand. Perhaps a clue lies in the fact that it was poor pitmen and steelworkers who cultured large succulent leeks for food and medicine before its rise to dizzy heights as a show plant.

Toiling underground every day led to many chest ailments, and consumption was a killer disease feared then as we fear cancer today. Leeks had been employed in cough remedies since the time of the Roman Emperor Nero. It was said that he used leeks to soften his voice; perhaps it helped to soothe his inflamed throat after the conflagration that destroyed part of Rome during his reign. There is little doubt that leeks played a part in treating those people burned while fighting the fire on the Seven Hills, as leeks are good treatment

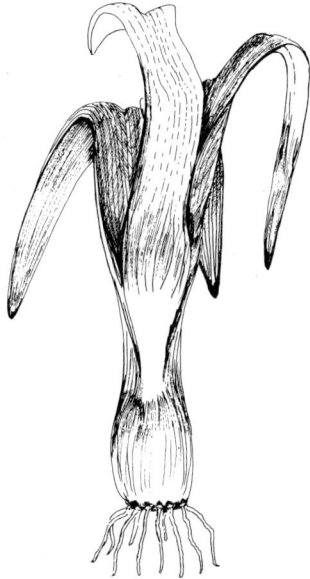

for minor burns; the juice is expressed from a whole plant and applied to the affected area as a salve. The Egyptians wrote of leeks as a burn treatment, regarding both juice and leaf as valid to soothe and heal damaged skin.

A cough syrup can be made by boiling three leeks in 150ml of water until soft, then pressing to extract the juice. Mix the juice, a quarter of the stock and 3 tablespoons of honey together, and take the mixture only when fresh. It is still a highly-thought-of cough remedy in some country districts.

Applications of leek juice and pulped leek to the skin in midsummer were used by country people when the attentions of harvest mites became unbearable. These tiny pests burrow into hair follicles and set up such irritation that victims can be driven half demented and frequently suffer secondary infection because of scratching which breaks the skin. The antiseptic and soothing properties of leek pulp will soon ease itching and help to disinfect the skin. This pulp is also recommended for wasp stings.

However, harvest mites were unlikely to trouble the poor workers who struggled deep underground in the mines of Britain's Midlands and the North-East. To them summer meant rampant intestinal infections caused by heat and poor sanitation. It was at this time of year that infant mortality through diarrhoea rose dramatically, and leeks were made into broth as a treatment for this dread malady. Stock prepared from leeks contains many minerals, and these helped to replace those lost through diarrhoea and sickness. The extra liquid was useful in this respect too. Leek's antiseptic properties allowed the gut flora to cope with the onslaught and helped reduce inflammation of the digestive system.

Lemon balm
(Melissa officinalis)
Family: LABIATAE

Sometimes called 'cure-all', there are a number of varieties of balm, of which the best-known is lemon

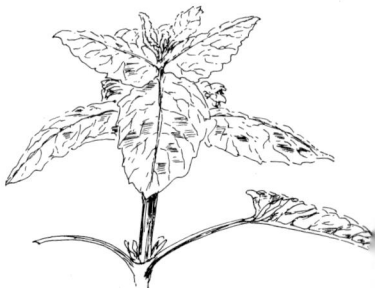

balm. The scientific name *Melissa* alludes to the honey collected in full measure by bees at the height of summer when balm flowers are in full bloom.

These flowers are the familiar labiate shape, small and white, and give a guide as to when the herb is ready for gathering. When the flowers are just about to open, the stems should be cut carefully with scissors at a leaf junction. The plant will quickly make new growth.

Stems, leaves and flowers should be made into bundles and hung, growing-point down, in the shade in an airy place. If the flowers have gone over, the pleasant lemony scent will not be retained, although balm's therapeutic value will remain unimpaired.

The very name 'balm' has become part of the English language, meaning something calming, soothing and beneficial, and there is every reason to believe that these properties are embodied by this plant so favoured by herbalists and laymen alike.

Arabs are so fond of the scent of balm that they preserve the fragrance in a perfumed oil for toilet use. Balm was said to form a vital ingredient in the elixir of life, and it features in remedies from the Middle East for treating epilepsy and mental illness.

An infusion can be made by steeping 2 cups of fresh flowering tips in 1 litre of boiling water for ten to fifteen minutes. When strained, this is said to be very good as a general tonic for digestion, colic, nervous indigestion and insomnia caused by heartburn. It is also recommended for menstrual cramps and as a pick-me-up for premenstrual tension.

Because considerable quantities of fresh plant are needed, your home stock of dried balm may be exhausted by the middle of winter, when a pick-me-up of balm tea would be much appreciated. In order not to deplete your supplies too quickly, spirit of balm can be obtained from herbalist shops. It is a complex mixture of many different herbs distilled after they have been mixed and macerated; not a practical proposition for home production.

Balm has the advantage of being very easy to grow in a sunny garden. However, it is invasive and should be planted in a container sunk into the soil. As with many of the mint family to which it belongs, the roots are surface propagating, and runners can be cut and replanted where required.

Lettuce
(Lactuca sativa)
Family: COMPOSITAE

When Beatrix Potter, the writer of children's stories, described lettuce as soporific in one of her tales about rabbits she was very near to the truth. I'm quite sure that with her knowledge of the countryside she was fully aware of the use to which an extract of this popular salad vegetable was put.

Lettuce's power to cool a fevered spirit was well documented in history, from the time the Emperor Diocletian told one of his advocates that he would rather tend his lettuces than take up the mantle of Emperor again, but there is some confusion as to which species of lettuce is referred to in many herbals.

Although normal salad lettuce has narcotic properties and seems to hold a popular place in herbal medicine as a narcotic, the plant from which the famous lettuce opium appears to be derived is actually a close relative called 'compass plant', or 'prickly lettuce' (*Lactuca virosa*) (pictured) which grows wild in Europe and when cut yields a milky secretion that hardens into a waxy brown compound with narcotic properties.

In Roman and Greek cultures lettuce was known as 'eunuch's plant' because it was supposed to reduce sexual desire, and the compound in the sap does appear to

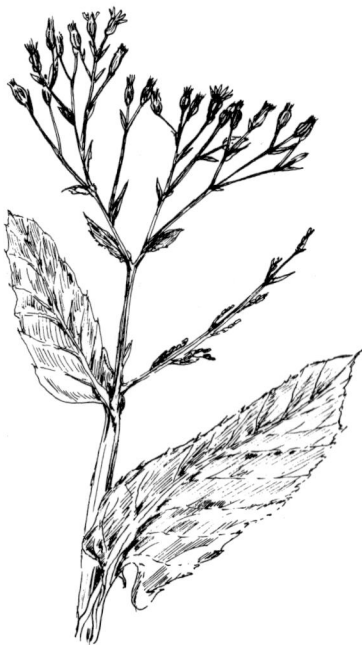

in the Doctrine of Signatures, because the oozing milky sap of lettuce was thought to resemble and therefore to be good for milk production. It is known that a mother's state of mind affects the flow of her milk, and perhaps the wet nurse felt so tranquil after her ration of lettuce that her milk flowed freely, but this must be pure speculation with little or no factual basis.

A soothing bedtime drink can be prepared by simmering a lettuce in 1 litre of water for half an hour. Strain off the juice and sweeten with honey. This is also useful in cases of bronchitis and diarrhoea.

Crushed lettuce leaves steeped in water are supposed to be a cold remedy, but though they have been used for this purpose for many years there is no evidence that they have any real value.

possess the ability to calm the sympathetic nervous system and also suppress sexual drive. The same virtue is shared by salad lettuce, but is offset by vitamin E in the leaves, thought to have a beneficial effect on sexual activity. Tales of its ability to quench the fires of lechery, supposedly inherited from both Greeks and Romans, were current well into the seventeenth century, and even now tincture of lettuce opium is recommended to cool sexual ardour.

In medieval times lettuce was given to wet nurses to increase the flow of milk. This idea had its roots

Lily of the valley
(Convallaria majalis)
Family: LILIACEAE

This rather attractive sweetly scented lily has been adopted into our regular garden flora with almost no alteration, but in the wild it favours old fissured limestone pavement such as is found in the Lake District.

The whole of the plant, from leaf to bulb, including the flowers, is poisonous. It contains a substance rather like digitalis, and although it is less powerful than foxglove

tions of an old dog-Latin name based in part on the name convallaria, and another corruption is thought to have led to the name 'male lily', from 'May lily'.

In the Middle Ages, herbalists appear to have considered it suitable for many ailments. For instance, Gerard thought that an extract in wine would restore speech to those who had been struck dumb, and also that a distillation of the flowers was excellent for improving eyesight.

In the midst of all the speculation and mysticism some genuine research was taking place, and several herbalists, but particularly Matthiolus, noticed that an extract of lily of the valley regularized heart rhythm and reduced dropsy following heart attacks; it is still used for this purpose today.

Because of the toxicity of this plant it should not be tampered with by amateurs, for quite small doses will lower blood pressure to a dangerous level. The onset of more serious effects are usually preceded by dizziness, with skin becoming cold and clammy. In severe cases there may be nausea followed by convulsion and heart failure.

Turning away from medicinal properties, lily of the valley leaves provide a dye apparently green in spring and early summer, changing to yellow when the leaves are gathered in late summer and early autumn.

However, it is not possible to gather this plant from the wild, for

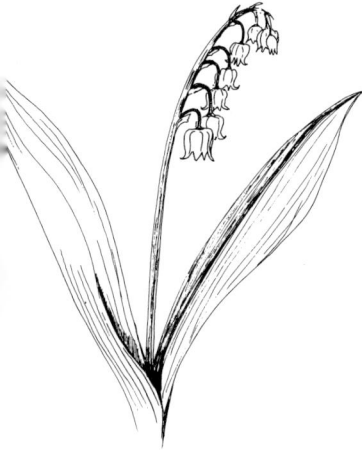

extract, an overdose can still cause the heart to lose rhythm and instigate a heart attack.

Despite its diminutive size, lily of the valley has attracted enough attention over the years to have gathered about itself a large number of country names. One of them, majalis (part of its scientific name), alludes to the month of May when it blooms, and the flowerspike with its bell-shaped delicate flowers has helped to connect it with the Christian church, for 'Mary's tears' is another common name.

In latter years of the Roman Empire it was known as 'glovewort' for its use in the care of hands, and in biblical vein again, the names 'Jacob's tears' and 'ladder to heaven' allude to the way the flowers form on one side of the stem. 'Lily constancy' and 'lirocon fancy' are thought to be corrup-

it is protected in many of its natural habitats in the United Kingdom, although not in the USA.

Lime/Linden tree
(Tilia europaea)
Family: TILIACEAE

Lime trees line many an avenue leading up to the stately homes of England. They can stand thirty metres or more tall and live for over a hundred years.

The wood is creamy and almost unrivalled as a timber for carving and turning, for purposes such as church sculpture and screens. Grinling Gibbons, a renowned woodcarver of the golden age of English church ornamentation, used limewood for all his most finely executed pieces, for when shaped with edged tools it takes a finish that remains sharp and crisp even after centuries; and although not durable when used out-of-doors, it is nonetheless highly prized.

In early spring the trees produce flowers with a strong smell of honey which bees find very attractive, but which can become infected with a fungal disease that kills bees in thousands. Nevertheless the flowers are a favourite with herbalists, although leaves and underbark have medicinal virtue too.

Dried flowers have to be treated carefully, as they quickly lose the volatile oil they contain. When prepared as a medicine for cold and flu symptoms care must be taken not to allow the water in which they are being infused to boil. If the temperature is too high the flowers will leach out a reddish dye which indicates that the active principles have been destroyed.

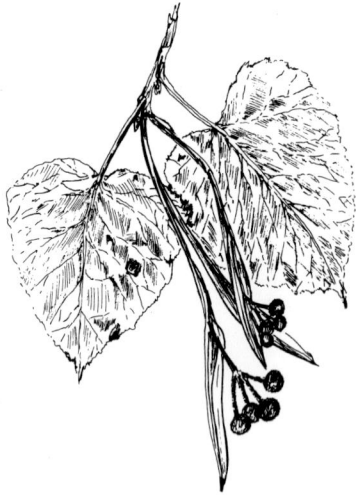

The volatile oil contained in the flowers and leaves is used to suppress nervous spasm and reduce discomfort caused by a cough; the mucilage soothes an inflamed throat lining to good effect.

Tinctures of lime flowers are prepared by herbalists and prescribed for nervous tension and vertigo, and have a beneficial effect on people suffering from high blood pressure. As a mild tranquillizer lime flowers have a great deal to recommend them. Lime bark, too, has its uses. When prepared as an infusion in very hot, not boiling, water, it can have a soothing effect on mild diarrhoea and in any case the liquid content is valuable to restore body fluid levels, always a problem with this dehydrating condition.

Liquorice
(Glycyrrhiza glabra)
Family: LEGUMINOSAE

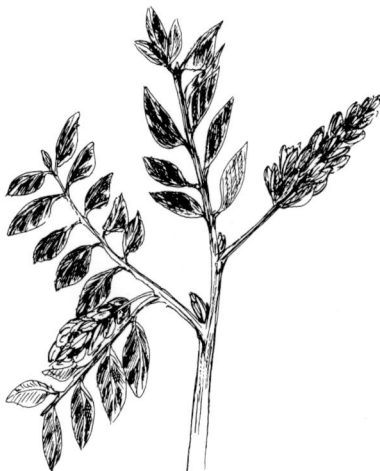

Most people are familiar with the taste of liquorice. It is one of the best-loved and oldest-established flavours in sweetmeats. In the earliest known records, inscribed on the Assyrian tablets over three thousand years ago, there are references to liquorice. Ancient Egyptians, Greeks, Romans, even the Hindus and Chinese valued its taste and medicinal properties.

English medieval monks cultivated the herb in a place that has become synonymous with liquorice, namely Pontefract. The monks made and sold small cakes of the black extract, and they are still very popular to this day, though not quite as the monks used to make them, for tastes and commercial pressures have far exceeded the capacity of the fields of Pontefract; in fact there is virtually no liquorice grown there today.

Liquorice is a member of the pea family, rather like a small bush with pink or blue flowers arranged in spires at the end of a short stem. The root is the valuable part, often reaching $1\frac{1}{2}$m in length, with the rest of the plant having no particular medicinal or culinary value. The thick woody rootstock is drawn by hand, a back-breaking job and highly labour-intensive, so there is little chance of it being grown in commercial quantities in the UK. Most of the liquorice root used in the British Isles is grown in Spain or the warmer regions of the Soviet Union.

The root is dried in the sun to produce a woody stick-like product which yields the sugary substance glycyrrhizin, probably fifty times sweeter than sugar. In the past this sweetness was added to mask unpleasant tastes in medicines.

Medicinally, liquorice seems to have been confined to using extracted juice for treating bronchitis and other chest infections, and there is good reason for believing that the active ingredients are fairly complex in their action upon the bronchial tract and do have real value as a constituent in cough remedies. Prepare as a tea by dissolving a teaspoon of finely ground liquorice powder in a cup of boiling water, and drink as required whilst still hot.

By the late Victorian era the middle classes, who seem to have been preoccupied with the regularity of their bowel movements, were taking powdered liquorice root as a laxative, and many children were forced to endure daily unwanted doses of liquorice.

It was during the Second World War that a Dutch doctor, F. E. Revers, noticed that some of his patients were recovering faster than usual from peptic ulcers and on inquiry found that a local stomach medicine they were taking contained large quantities of liquorice. On further investigation he discovered that in massive doses the powdered extract did have a healing effect on ulcers, but that it had side-effects too, causing higher-than-normal blood pressure and in some cases inducing dropsy, which set back what had looked like a promising line of research. It was only much later that he was able to report that an extracted active ingredient (since called carbenoxolone) had a significant cortisone-like ability to heal stomach ulcers – a far cry from the days when Greek warriors

chewed liquorice to allay the pangs of thirst and Roman legions were issued it as part of their rations.

Of course, any treatment for stomach ulcers is only sensible if undertaken with the full knowledge of your medical adviser, who will have made a diagnosis of your condition.

Extracts of liquorice are available from herbalists and pharmacists, and the root can often be obtained from health food stores and some chemists.

Mallow, marsh
(Althaea officinalis)
Family: MALVACEAE

USA: English mallow

Certain plants possess names, familiar in other contexts, and this makes it difficult to envisage them in their plant form. Such a one is marsh mallow. In the mind's eye the name conjures up a vision of a soft pink-and-white foaming confection, very sweet and made from sugar, gelatine and rose water.

The root does bear a passing, but rather tenuous, resemblance to the sweet in that it is rich in sugar and mucilage and sickly in taste; in the past it was used as an ingredient in sweetmeats, but now the only connection is in the name.

Before changes in agriculture made the pond and damp meadow a thing of the past, marsh mallow was a reasonably common plant

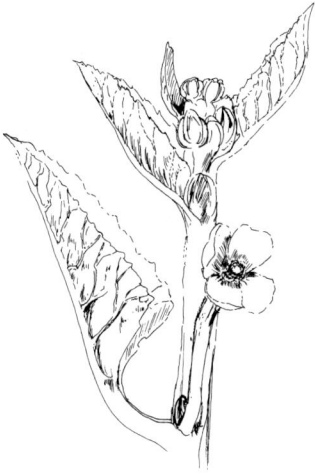

Originally it is thought to have been an import from China, where no doubt its medicinal virtues were well known. It was mentioned by the Greeks in their herbals, where they recommended the root and a tea made from the dried leaves as a remedy for intestinal troubles. The Romans refined its use and it was widely employed both as a laxative and to treat diarrhoea, especially in children.

found by the streamside and at the freshwater end of estuaries in southern England. A plant of neutral-to-alkaline habitat, it grows best in the south and south-east, but can be grown in gardens near a pond or actually in a water garden.

There are several members of the mallow family, but marsh mallow is the main medicinal herb in the group carrying the suffix *officinalis*. A large spreading bushy plant, it grows to a height of 1m. The lobed serrated-edged leaves are downy on the underside and greenish-grey in colour. Arranged on alternate sides of the stem, the single leaf carries the flower buds at the base where it joins the stem. The flowers, a lovely pale pink and rather showy, have a raised central portion; this is altogether a very attractive plant.

The root and, to a lesser extent, the leaves, contain large amounts of mucilage, and Culpeper, who was familiar enough with the healing virtues of mallow, noted that the crushed root when steeped in water produced so much mucilage that the water became viscous, almost like jelly. The Romans and herbalists of the Middle Ages used marsh mallow as an expectorant for chest ailments, for which it was very effective, as apart from the copious mucilage the active ingredients of the leaf and root consist of a volatile oil and tannin.

The grated root has been employed for centuries as a poultice for wounds and burns and as a field dressing. There are a number of recipes for poultices containing mallow, and all of them appear to be quite effective. However, some of them sound pleasanter than others, especially fresh grated root mixed with honey.

For cuts and minor burns a recommended poultice can be made as follows. Grate the fresh root into a bowl and crush until it becomes a thick paste, then add

1 tablespoon of honey. This makes an ideal ointment to apply to open wounds. If honey is not used, the crushed root should be allowed to soak for approximately 1 hour in a little boiled water, then brought to boiling point in order to kill any bacteria.

Two important points to remember when using herbal plasters are absolute cleanliness in the preparation, and fresh ingredients and mixture for each application. There is always the possibility of introducing bacteria into a wound through poor hygiene. This is where honey is excellent, for it is a natural inhibitor of the growth of micro-organisms.

When treating a boil, apply the same recipe after warming the ointment on a plate over hot water.

The Romanies, experts at using natural medicines, still eat the shoots and tips of marsh mallow as a vegetable. Eaten raw they are a natural indigestion preventative. The Romans, too, ate the shoots, and the poet Horace stated publicly that he lived on a diet of which mallow played a major part. In the relief of indigestion and constipation the mucilage has a lubricating effect and produces bulk.

A tea made from the leaves and flowers has been used for centuries to relieve the symptoms of cystitis, and the most popular recipe seems to be as follows: 30g of dried leaves and flowers steeped in 1 litre of cold water for 10 minutes, brought to the boil for a further 3 minutes, and allowed to cool. One cupful of the tea should be taken four times a day before meals.

Mallow, common
(Malva sylvestris)
Family: MALVACEAE

USA: mallow

Common mallow was thought better for relieving skin irritations than marsh mallow, and it has the advantage of being a more easily available plant. It is a common roadside weed, but because of its habitat, any plants to be employed for medicinal purposes should be gathered as far away from traffic contamination as possible. The low-growing crinkled foliage is a ready trap for heavy metal contaminants.

Unlike marsh mallow, which is showy and immediately noticeable, common mallow is more of a spreading plant. The flowers have the attractive raised centre of all the family malva, but are small and a soft bluish-pink in colour. The seed cases are button-shaped and hard, and can be collected and crushed to make a skin lotion. 30g of seeds crushed in 1 litre of water, brought to the boil and allowed to cool, will make a good lotion for the relief of dry, itching skin, and has been used to help eczema sufferers. As with all allergic skin conditions, a test should be made on a small area of unaffected skin to see if there are any adverse reactions.

In the past mallow flowers were chewed to relieve toothache and sore gums, and the lobed leaves were used in much the same way as marsh mallow. The general effect of common mallow is gently purgative, and it is said to be an excellent treatment for all mild gastric upsets. In the Middle Ages it was a much valued herb.

It can be cultivated easily, but is invasive and once established can take over the garden unless drastically controlled.

Mallow, musk
(Malva moschata)
Family: MALVACEAE

This plant shares all the properties of its two cousins, marsh mallow and common mallow. It is the most beautiful of the wild mallows, and the fine cut leaves and large showy pink flowers are an asset to any wild garden or woodside walk.

A plant that prefers alkaline soil, it can be found in the south-east of England in disused chalk quarries where there has been a considerable recolonization of brush and hawthorn and where blackberries have sheltered the plants in their early growing stages. It was introduced to north America possibly as early as the seventeenth century.

Musk mallow is the one most highly recommended for cough remedies and poultices. Only the leaves and flowers are used for the cough remedy. 50g of dried leaf and flower mixture are steeped in 1 litre of boiled water, brought back to the boil and simmered for 5 minutes. The cooled tea is sweetened with honey and taken as required. Its purgative effect is not quite as strong as that of marsh or common mallow.

Mallow root is thick and fleshy and can be dried in readiness for future use (this applies to marsh, common and musk mallow). The mucilage attracts water, so it must be completely dried before storage, or mould will form. Cleanliness is vital, and the root should be scrubbed to remove all dirt and any small stones. Best of all is to partly dry and grate it very finely, then dry again in an airing cupboard or some similar area. Mucilage will pick up smells and fix them, so take care not to prepare the root where it's likely to come into contact with strong odours. To ensure that the root remains uncontaminated, store in an airtight container.

Leaves and flowers should be dried in a warm place too, preferably on a muslin screen. This will allow rapid drying that does not destroy either their colour or potency. When dry, crush them and store in dark airtight glass containers where they will keep for a considerable period of time.

All species of mallow root can be reconstituted for poultices by soaking 50g of dried grated root in

20ml of boiled water for an hour. Work this into a paste for a cool boil plaster, or add a little honey for use as a treatment for spots.

And remember that in the field the herb gatherer may well be stung by a bee or wasp. The leaves of all species of mallow can be crushed and rubbed on the skin to reduce inflammation.

Marigold
(Calendula officinalis)
Family: COMPOSITAE

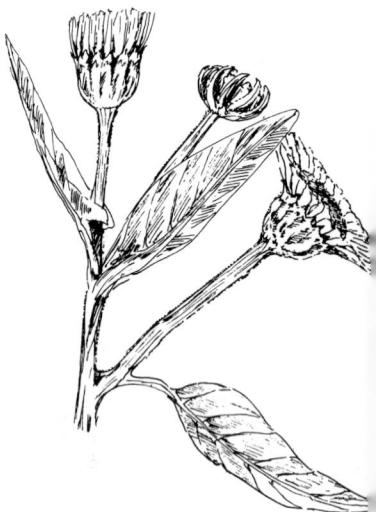

Once held in contempt by keen gardeners who considered it almost a weed, this free-flowering member of the daisy family is hard to overlook. It will flower in the countryside, which has led to its being confused with the small and now relatively rare corn marigold (*Chrysanthemum segetum*).

It is thought that marigolds originated in the East and were brought, along with spices and silks, from Asia, especially India, where they are sacred and it is the custom for flowerheads to be strung in garlands at Hindu shrines.

The Romans adopted the dried petals as a substitute for saffron, which has always been an expensive colouring material. Marigold flower petals are dried by arranging them on blotting paper in a warm shady place. When quite dry, crush and store in dark-glass bottles until required.

For colouring rice, a teaspoon of dried flowers is added to the cooking water at the same time as the rice. The petals will not only lend a light golden colour to the grains, they will also give a sharp resinous tang which overlays the blandness of the rice.

Actually it was to treat the after-effects of cooking that marigold flowers were most frequently used in the past. A popular remedy for indigestion was an infusion of marigold made with a handful of dried flowers to 1 litre of boiling water. Steep for 10 minutes, then drink a cupful at a time until the symptoms subside. A tincture of marigold is available from herbal suppliers, and can also be used for digestive disorders and to ease painful menstrual periods, although this latter action is now in doubt.

Externally, marigolds can help heal cuts and abrasions. Prepare an infusion of fresh flowers and apply to the wound.

The fleshy leaves of marigold are edible, too, and are often put into salads in Mediterranean regions and said to be quite palatable. Desert tribesmen in the Middle East used the flower heads in a strengthening medicine for their stallions and brood mares. They believed that it made their offspring stronger and more fleet of foot.

It's not easy to gather and dry marigold petals, and any which are discoloured should be thrown out, for they will have a bitter taste.

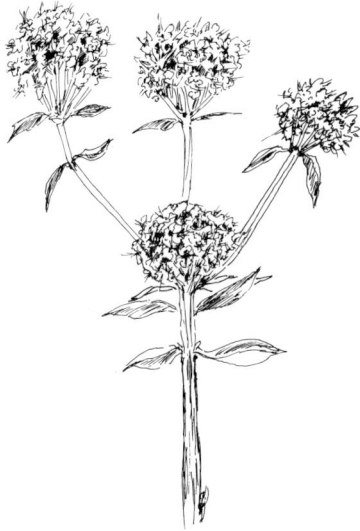

Marjoram
(Origanum vulgare)
Family: LABIATAE

USA: sweet marjoram

A great many of the most useful herbs have a variety of common names, but there are exceptions to every rule, and the immensely valuable herb marjoram must be one as there are virtually no other names attributed to it.

The terms 'pot marjoram', 'common marjoram', and 'sweet marjoram' are all applied to the culinary variety of this plant (*Origanum marjorana*). All over the land there are kitchen spice racks containing this herb. Many a jar filled with unhealthy-looking straw-coloured chaff-like stuff is taken down and used as a flavouring only once in a while. Yet there are few herbs more beneficial, either in cooking or for relieving head-cold symptoms.

Although the two varieties of marjoram mentioned are almost identical to look at, wild marjoram is the more valuable for its medicinal properties. It contains more of the aromatic oil thymol than is found in the cultivated variety.

This herb is steeped in legend. The Greeks planted marjoram on the tombs of their dead to give departing spirits peace and comfort, but for the living too it has endless uses: for cold and cough symptoms, lotions for sickly children, skin complaints, etc.

In the past marjoram was a very common plant in the southern half of the country, but changes in our countryside, the use of weed-killers, and the ploughing and mowing of banks and rough corners have made it far less common. Nevertheless it is an easy plant to grow both from seeds and cuttings, and is available from nurseries and seedsmen. It does require a very sunny, well-drained bank to do really well. It is most popular with bees during the flowering season in late July and early August.

The dust inhaled at harvest-time from cereal crops has long been known to cause a fungal disease known as 'farmer's lung', which if untreated results in endless problems. Flowering marjoram was formerly taken as a drink and an inhalation to reduce tightness in the chest, and the antiseptic effect of thymol in the steam during inhalation must have given considerable relief. Now there are far more effective ways of dealing with farmer's lung, but the antispasmodic effect of the herb still holds good.

For common cold symptoms the recommended recipe is as follows. Take 2 tablespoons of dried marjoram flowerheads, pour on 1 pint of boiling water, cover with a saucer and allow to stand for at least 10 minutes. Then add a tablespoon of honey and the juice of 1 lemon. Stir until the honey has dissolved, as this has the added benefit of leaching out more of the active ingredient. Strain and drink whilst hot. This mixture has a pleasant flavour and is also good for sore throats caused by a stuffy nose. Brandy or whisky may be added, and although this has little effect on the cold it can have a considerable effect on the sufferer!

Marjoram tea should always be freshly made and taken as a temporary measure. It should not be used to treat a persistent cough, and proper medical attention should be sought if symptoms do not abate after several days.

Marsh woundwort
(Stachys palustris)
Family: LABIATAE

Our grandfathers relied on tools of ferocious sharpness and lethal design, which must have caused many cuts and abrasions in their daily lives. Hedgers in particular needed a safe, easily available remedy for the frequent accidents that occurred during the course of their work. This is how members of the stachys family of woundworts became popular as a form of emergency treatment in the field and hedge bottom.

At that time, before antibiotics such as penicillin were developed, the threat of blood poisoning was an ever-present danger to those who worked on the land and in factories, for often their resistance to infection was low through poverty, overwork and poor diet.

Until the First World War conflict between armies was usually

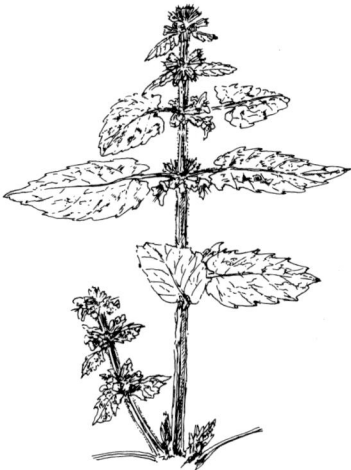

bleeding and promote healing, but this is only an emergency measure until a sterile dressing can be procured.

Meadowsweet
(Filipendula ulmaria)
Family: ROSACEAE

USA: meadowsweet, my lady's bett, queen of the meadow

Meadowsweet, as its name suggests, is a plant of open fields and meadows, a vanishing habitat in the British Isles, but there are still a few places in Dorset and Devon where fields rich with the scent of this tall stately plant can be found.

Not for nothing was the suffix 'sweet' added to its name. The scent of these flowers is not easily forgotten when inhaled on warm summer evenings. Meadowsweet also has many practical uses.

The leaves, which resemble those of ground elder in shape and elm in texture, precede the tall flowering spikes which open into an umbrella of creamy flowers cascading down the stem as the plant matures.

The plants grow to varying heights, depending on soil conditions and the amount of sun they get. Those growing on the shady side of a hedge will reach 1m in height, and those opening their flowers on the sunward side will reach a full 1½m before setting seeds.

Long before modern painkillers were discovered meadowsweet

carried on in a close-combat situation. After the musketry or archers had played their part, there was hand-to-hand fighting with sharp-edged weapons, and the wounds inflicted were deadly, killing through shock or loss of blood, or by disablement and subsequent death through infection. The death rate of foot soldiers and officers alike was appalling. A relatively minor injury almost always led to secondary infection.

For these reasons, woundwort was held in high regard. It was also known as 'Saracen's consound', a reference to its use in the field of battle.

Administer this plant by steeping a handful of dried woundwort in 1 litre of boiling water; use this to bathe an infected area. Pounded fresh plant placed on a cut will stay

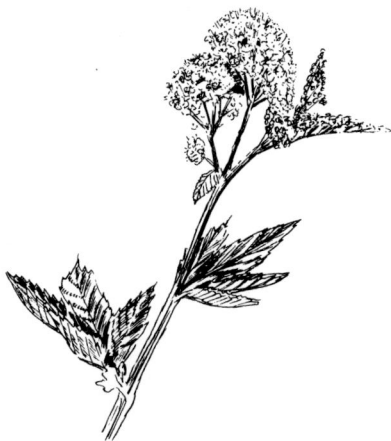

was administered to soothe aching heads and joints.

When crushed, the flowers give off a characteristic odour of salicylic aldehyde, and it is this chemical compound which led to the discovery of synthesized aspirin. The route taken by chemists to arrive at the compound now known as aspirin was tortuous indeed.

In 1838 the Italian chemist Raffaele Piria discovered that oxydized salicylic aldehyde yielded salicylic acid, and by 1853 another chemist, Strasbourg-based Charles Frédéric Gerhardt, was using this compound to produce acetyl-salicylic acid, which became known as aspirin. This name has a direct connection with meadowsweet as a corruption of the scientific name spirea.

Aspirin is commonly used for relieving pain and inflammation, and after many years of research it has been found that few other drugs give such considerable relief from arthritis and rheumatism as the humble aspirin. Recently it has been found that patients who have suffered coronary artery disease can also benefit from treatment with aspirin.

It does have some side-effects, however, and some people cannot tolerate the compound. It can cause severe bleeding from the stomach lining, and many people have some form of stomach upset after prolonged use.

The active ingredients of meadowsweet are buffered to some extent, seeming not to possess the side-effects of the refined constituent chemicals. Consequently, infusions of meadowsweet flowers and leaf can be helpful in relieving head pains and mild rheumatic conditions where side-effects might be a problem, and have now even been successfully used to treat inflammation of the stomach lining.

A high level of tannin is found in the root, which makes it a handy wound dressing, and indeed infusions of the whole plant are applied to promote healing of severe grazes and to reduce discomfort from bruises and sprains.

In the past meadowsweet was used for gout, and it seems the active ingredients in the plant do assist in removing the uric acid crystals found in the joints of people who suffer from this agonizing condition.

Although meadowsweet is declining rapidly from loss of

habitat in the wild, it can be obtained from herbalists everywhere as a prepared tincture, so there is little point in collecting it from the countryside yourself and perhaps diminishing it still further.

Melilot
(Melilotus officinalis)
Family: LEGUMINOSAE

Everything about melilot is impressive. The golden-yellow spires of flowers, the scent of honey that so attracts bees, and the bright-green foliage. There is little wonder Ancient Egyptians used it as a symbol of life. They considered it a charm against the forces of darkness, and as well as using it in treatments for earache and bruises they incorporated it in many other potent medicines. In the past it was compounded in a remedy for drunkenness, especially to 'calm the rage' of extreme intoxication.

So widely administered by physicians in the Middle Ages was it that it gained the name 'king's clover', and was added to so many potions purporting to cure all ills that eventually it fell from favour. This is unfortunate, for it does have considerable worth as a medicinal herb.

The dried flowering tips have a sweet smell of coumarin, and prepared as an infusion (a handful of dried tips in 1 litre of boiling water), they taste quite pleasant. Care should be taken when drying this plant, however, as fermentation can produce a poisonous product called dicoumarol, which inhibits the absorption of vitamin K. It is better to use the herb fresh.

Melilot's properties are varied. Calming the nervous system and stomach is one, especially in cases

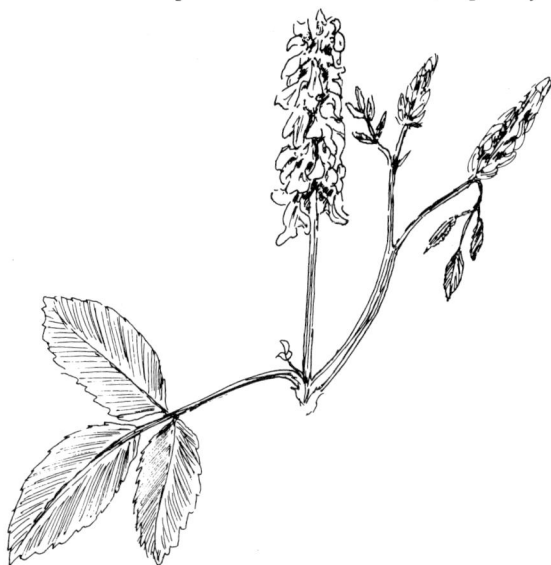

of nervous indigestion, and the same infusion as above will relieve discomfort caused by menstrual cramps. It has been said that a tea made with melilot tips in boiling water is very beneficial in treating premenstrual tension.

Milk thistle
(Silybum marianum)
Family: COMPOSITAE

As a boy I can remember going out with a small scythe into the fields surrounding my home in Devon to cut docks and thistles so they wouldn't spring up the following year. It was a never-ending task, for the multitude of seeds shed by one clump of thistle would soon repopulate the area that had been cleared.

The name 'milk thistle' has a biblical significance. It was said to have grown up where a drop of milk had fallen from the breast of the Virgin Mary as she gathered food for her donkey. A pretty story, and it's easy to see how the connection came about, for the sap of this thistle is white and milky, although it quickly curdles and coagulates to a brown latex-like resin with certain weak narcotic properties similar to lettuce opium.

It has been misnamed in various parts of Europe, often being confused with the common dark green thistle (*Cirsium arvense*) and the spear thistle (*Cirsium vulgare*). However, the leaves are the telling feature. They are green, veined

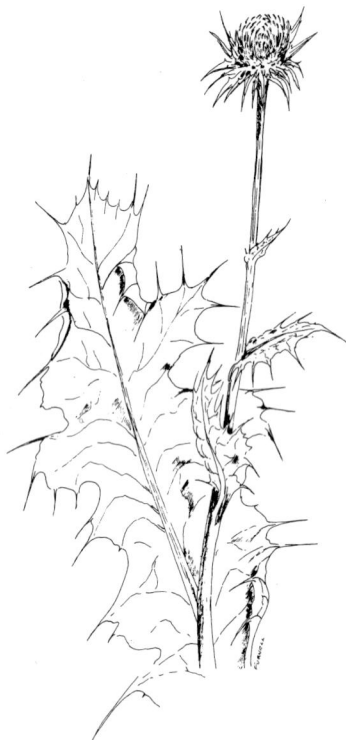

with yellowish white – a very attractive combination.

The flowerhead is typical of thistle, surrounded by a crown of thorns just below the purple composite head of flowers. This may well have added to its biblical associations.

It has been suggested that the heads were dried and used as carding tools or combs for wool prior to spinning, but the shape of the thistle head would have resulted in a very crude carding process; most likely the true teasel (*Dipsacus fullonum*) was the plant used.

In medicine, milk thistle is mainly employed externally, the soft leaves being stripped of prickles and the whole bruised leaf bound over a persistent sore or a place which is slow to heal, especially one that has been infected. The plaster of leaves should be changed frequently. As you may imagine, this remedy comes from the Middle East where high temperatures and flies that reinfect wounds tend to cause deep sores that are slow to heal; the Arabs put great store in this plant for treating epilepsy and schizophrenia too.

The leaves are rich in minerals such as calcium and are recommended for certain deficiency diseases like rickets. They also contain vitamin C, which was used to heal scurvy. The seeds, gathered before they open fully, were once considered to have great value in treating rabies; though we know today that this disease is so severe as to be untreatable without the help of modern drugs and vaccines.

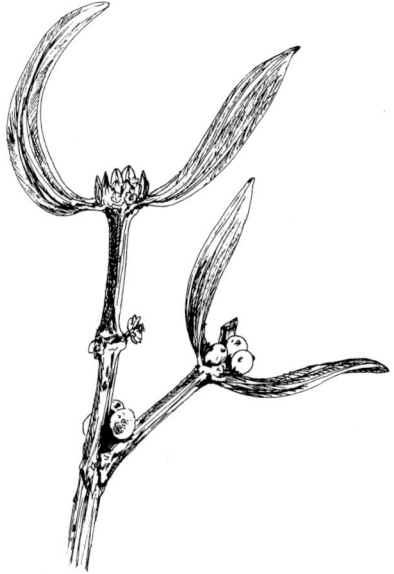

Mistletoe

(Viscum album)
Family: LORANTHACEAE

This plant has filled a ceremonial role in these islands for many thousands of years. Armsful of mistletoe are gathered during December to decorate our houses, but these days we use shears, not a golden sickle as the Druids did.

Druids thought that mistletoe could confer eternal life, which is not surprising, for it is green and vigorous when the rest of nature is asleep. They revered this plant because it appeared to spring from living trees unaided by seeds or soil, especially apple and pear trees, which were also considered by the Druids to have spiritual qualities.

They used it in their most solemn rituals and called it the immortal, the plant that heals all ills. At the end of their great rituals to mark the beginning of spring and coming of winter, Druid priests gathered sprigs of mistletoe with a golden sickle, and these sprigs were given to their followers to wear as amulets and charms against illness and evil spirits. It was the practice of hanging a sprig of mistletoe at the door as a talisman that formed the basis of our modern-day Yuletide custom of kissing under the mistletoe.

This strange plant with its sticky yellow berries and pallid leaves was not only revered in England. At the time of the Druids ancient Teuton tribes who occupied what we now call Germany believed mistletoe made them invincible in battle. These warlike tribesmen had such faith in its virtues that it led them to great victories over other tribes and clans in Europe. The Teutons also thought the berries would restore fertility to their farm animals.

Belief in the power of mistletoe was also strong in parts of Austria. A sprig of mistletoe over the bedroom door was said to render sleepers safe from nightmares, and nearer to home a Welsh maiden would sleep with a sprig of mistletoe under her pillow in the hope of dreaming of her future husband, and seeing his face.

Yet on a more practical level mistletoe leaves have always been used medicinally, mostly as a treatment for high blood pressure and heart ailments, and there is some medical support for its use as an anti-spasmodic. It was the standard country herbal remedy for convulsions caused by epilepsy.

Head pains are often a symptom of high blood pressure, and mistletoe employed as a treatment for migraine probably goes hand-in-hand with its use for this condition. However, it is extremely unwise and can be dangerous to attempt to treat hypertension (high blood pressure) with herbal medicines without first establishing the true cause. Under no circumstances should you treat yourself or anyone else unless you are qualified to do so or have been instructed by a properly qualified person. For instance, although mistletoe is found in a variety of remedies and in the past was widely recommended for its efficacy in reducing whooping cough symptoms in small children, children are at risk if they consume the berries, which are not unpalatable because of their sugar content. These berries are in fact highly poisonous; only the leaves are used medicinally, and even then only in moderation.

Mouse-ear hawkweed
(Hieracium pilosella)
Family: COMPOSITAE

It's not easy to see how this plant, resembling a cross between a thistle and a dandelion, could possibly have been so named. According to the *Dictionary of English Plant Names*, 'hawkweed' derives from a sixteenth-century Greek

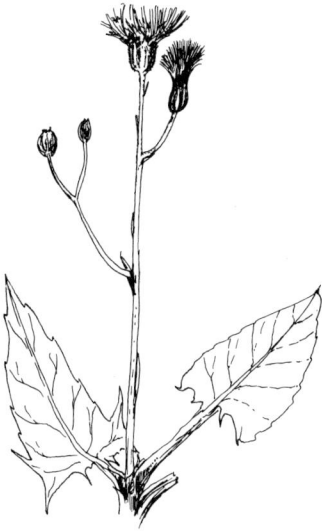

hawkweed flowers, which are the same bright yellow as dandelions – indeed, the two plants belong to the same family.

Like the dandelion, hawkweed has a long and illustrious history as a useful herb. Peasant farmers in Britain and Europe had a saying 'God puts the cure beside the ill', and this is often found to be true; such plants as docks and stinging nettles are usually found growing together, and dock leaves, when rubbed on skin freshly stung by nettles, do seem to relieve the irritation somewhat.

The same applies to hawkweed, but with veterinary connotations, for the plant was thought to be a remedy for abortion in cattle and it often grows near paths frequented by cows. Experiments have shown that a solution of the latex-like juice from the stems mixed with water has a mild antibiotic effect on the bacteria which can cause these ills in livestock.

On the Continent, where herbal medicine is held in higher regard than in Britain, it is prescribed to reduce fevers by administering the bitter-tasting juice in a draught of wine. Fresh plants should be used.

One school of thought in herbal circles is promoting hawkweed extract as a treatment for hardening of the arteries, but there seems to be little real evidence to support this. Nevertheless, there is often a grain of truth hidden away in many of the old wives' tales, and there are a number of references in ancient herbals to hawkweed for

translation. The scholar Turner, who translated the *Hieracion* of Pliny, found the connection in the Greek word for a hawk, *hierax*. It was said that birds of prey used to pull this plant out of the ground and smear it on their eyes to cure poor sight, but it transpires that the plant Pliny referred to is not hawkweed as we know it, but a related plant found in Greece.

The connection with hawks has its own mythology in English country folklore, and though the two myths are alike in their conclusions they have arisen separately. Old English folklore suggests that the plant received its name because sparrow-hawks and goshawks, both yellow-eyed birds of prey, kept the colouring of the iris by anointing their eyes with

heart ailments. Dropsy was associated with heart conditions, and as hawkweed is a diuretic it was adopted for the relief of that illness.

The white latex sap was administered by herbalists who followed the Doctrine of Signatures for treating breast congestion, because the sap resembled milk. Culpeper also recommended it for ulcers.

Hawkweed does not appear to have found as much favour in Britain as on the Continent, and it could well be that there is more value in this weed of the fields than we yet realize.

Mugwort

(Artemisia vulgaris)
Family: COMPOSITAE

USA: artemisia, mugwort

Mugwort is well known as a remedy for menstrual disorders, and there are many references to it in sixteenth- and seventeenth-century herbals. Culpeper ascribed the plant to the influence of Venus, and considered it helpful for all female disorders. Gerard thought it very good for palsy, and the juice was recommended for expelling worms in children and curing fits.

The Greeks had a great deal of faith in mugwort as a 'bringer of good health' and as a remedy for travel weariness. Pliny is said to have advised that a sprig of this herb be tied to travellers' waistbands to prevent them from feeling

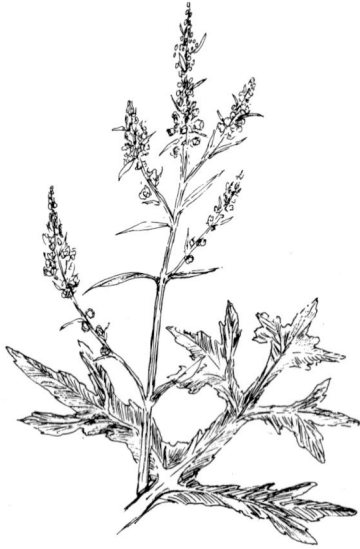

tired, a theme carried on by the Germans, who hung a spray of mugwort over the door to save the house from a multitude of ills.

In England the practice was to wear a sprig of mugwort in your belt on Midsummer's Day. When fires were lit in the evening the Midsummer revellers threw their sprigs of mugwort into the fire; with them went all the ills of the year to come.

This common wayside plant has always been surrounded by this kind of folklore. At one time it was thought that carrying a sprig of mugwort kept stinging and poisonous creatures at bay, and that wearers would be protected from anyone who wished them ill by poison.

However, although mugwort is

still used by some herbalists for relieving menstrual disorders, it does contain several compounds that can be harmful and should not be taken during pregnancy or without proper supervision. It is a very common plant and easily obtained, but prolonged use can lead to a build-up of these compounds, which are thought to be injurious to the central nervous system.

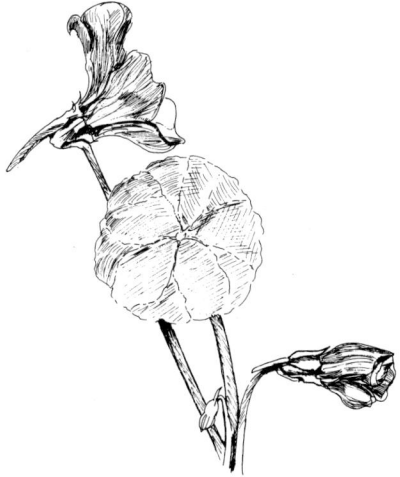

Nasturtium
(Tropaeolum majus)
Family: CRUCIFERAE

Nasturtiums will grow anywhere. Originally a plant of the high Andes in Central America, they were brought to Europe by marauding Conquistadors as a symbol of victory and gold.

The flower is spurred, and similar in shape to a Greek warrior's helmet, with the leaves having a passing resemblance to a Greek shield; its scientific name refers to the trophies of helm and shield which Greeks used to adorn triumphal arches.

Andean air must have an excellent effect on nasturtiums, for in their native land they are perennial, whereas in less favoured climes such as Europe they feature as annuals, being mainly propagated by the caper-like seeds that follow the flowers.

The flowers have a peculiar quality in that under certain conditions of humidity and temperature they emit a small spark of fire between stamen and style. It appears that this phenomenon is due to a high phosphorus content in the flower. That nasturtium is associated with fire is apt, for both seeds and leaves can have an extremely hot taste. In the seventeenth century they were used as capers in pickling, and in some country districts of south-western England and central France nasturtium seeds are still pickled in vinegar as a condiment.

The beautiful flower grows on a stalk a little too short to be really useful for decoration, and in the early days of the plant's European history its flowers were not valued at all except by bumblebees, who found the nectary much to their liking. The leaves were eaten in salads, for they are piquant and add a peppery flavour to lettuce which otherwise can be rather bland.

When used medicinally to reduce stomach infections it has the benefit of not causing colic, despite its high sulphur content, and in Germany it has been called the flower of love because of its supposed aphrodisiac properties. However, its value as a treatment for chest infections is more tangible than any supposed virtue as a plant of love.

Its use as a hair treatment is also widespread, and a tonic rub may be made from a few handfuls of nasturtium plant, nettle leaves and a small handful of box leaves. Crush and place in a screw-top jar with a quarter of a pint of vodka or aquavit. The whole should be allowed to soak for two weeks, when the alcohol, which will have absorbed the essential properties of the plants, should be strained off. A small amount massaged into the scalp promotes a brisk circulation.

This lotion may be scented by adding a teaspoonful of crushed rosemary leaves, preferably fresh, and a similar quantity of fresh lavender flower heads during the second week of its preparation. Being alcoholic, it will keep for some time.

Nettle
(Urtica dioica)
Family: URTICACEAE

USA: stinging nettle

Nettles are born colonizers and survivors. They are common wherever there is disturbed ground and where man has set up home.

They feature frequently in British and north American folklore as medicinal plants, and their stinging foliage has long been much respected. However, some foreign species, especially those in India and Africa, are virulent in their power. The poison in the fine hollow leaf hairs is formic acid, the same acid used by ants to protect themselves from attack, and this sets up intense irritation when the skin is pierced.

The old country treatment for nettle stings was to rub large crushed dock leaves over an affected area, and if this is carried out soon enough any stinging and subsequent irritation does subside. Crushed nettle itself also has the power to alleviate nettle stings fairly quickly.

Because they are so common and difficult to handle, nettles are neglected both as food and as medicinal plants. Cooking removes the formic acid and softens the stinging organs on the leaves, which can then be eaten in much the same way as spinach. They have a pleasant flavour and are excellent with lemon juice and a little butter.

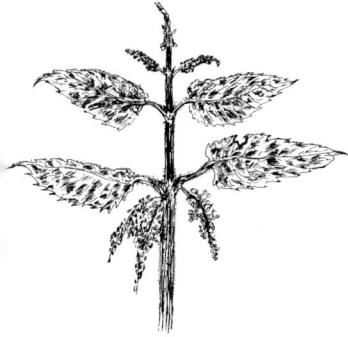

Young nettles are rich in vitamin C and iron in usable quantities, as well as many other minerals and trace elements.

The name 'nettle' is believed to derive from the old English *netele*, meaning 'to twist', and possibly referring to the fact that nettle was an ancient textile plant.

Nettles have been used by man for thousands of years as food and as a source of fibre for fabric. When nettle stems are retted, that is, treated with water to break down the stems, a fibre very similar to flax is produced. From this fibre a type of linen fabric can be woven, and samples of actual cloth woven from nettles have been found covering the remains of Bronze Age sacrificial victims in Danish peat bogs. The fabric has survived so well that the methods of spinning and weaving can be reproduced today.

The stinging power of nettles has been used to alleviate pain in certain rheumatic conditions. An application of nettles over an affected area seems to short-circuit the body's pain response, and the discomfort from the nettle stings is offset by a reduction in joint pains. However, I should think that the long-term skin irritation of repeated nettle applications would outweigh any relief gained.

The idea behind it would appear similar to a rather painful and dangerous method used by some alternative practitioners of bee-sting therapy, which can provoke an allergic response in some patients that might lead to death.

In homoeopathic medicine nettles are used for bruises, chicken-pox, gout, and even as a remedy for nettle-rash! In older herbals Gerard attributes to nettles the power to allay the effects of all manner of poisons, including mercuric compounds, but modern medicinal uses are more concerned with the plant as a tonic, with seeds and stems being boiled in a little water for 10 minutes then drunk to relieve coughs and colds.

Nettle beer or tea made from a mixture of dried leaves, flowers and seeds is well known as a tonic, and it does have diuretic properties as well as being mildly astringent.

A lotion for mild burns is prepared by pouring a cup of boiling water onto a tablespoon of dried nettle leaves and allowing to cool. This is only of use if absolutely fresh, as the possibility of secondary infection with burns is always to be borne in mind.

Old man's beard

(Clematis vitalba)
Family: RANUNCULACEAE

USA: clematis, traveller's joy

In days gone by the flowers and fruiting bodies of this climbing plant were a very familiar sight in the English countryside, and other names include 'traveller's joy' and, less understandably, 'virgin's bower'.

At first sight it would appear to be a member of the vine family, but in fact it is more closely related to buttercups than grapes.

The leaves are typical of a climber, having the shape of vine or hop to catch the sun even in a shaded environment and providing the necessary fuel for the plant to climb to the daylight. The flowers are fairly insignificant, and are often overlooked altogether. It is the seed heads which follow after the flowers that gave the plant its name of 'old man's beard'. They burst from the cases in a flurry of grey down which has a remarkable resemblance to a beard.

This material is the means whereby the plant transports its seed on the wind to hedgerow and woods. It is not like thistledown, because it remains on the bine for some time, and hedges where it is common can be covered with so many seed-capsule fronds that the whole hedge is obscured by a mass of grey fluff.

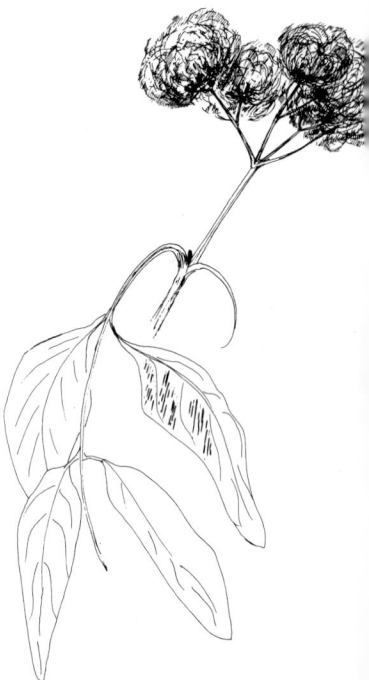

The name 'traveller's joy' came about because travellers picked tips and young leaves to make into a refreshing tea, and there are records of travellers, especially the drovers who roamed the length and breadth of Britain, plucking young fronds to add to their bottles of ale.

Restorative properties contained in this plant have been used as a stimulant for travel weariness for centuries, and it is likely pilgrims gathered it for this purpose and also to prepare a poultice for tired feet. They may also have steeped their headcloths in an infusion of traveller's joy to relieve headaches caused by tired eyes and general fatigue.

A lotion prepared by boiling a handful of tips in 1 litre of water for 10 minutes was found excellent as a wayside treatment for saddle-sores, both for man and beast, and blisters caused by ill-fitting sandals and uneven dusty roads were also relieved.

The rigours of journeying two and three centuries ago had to be experienced to be believed. Flies and clegs that bit travellers and their animals caused infected sores that were slow to heal in the heat and dust of a pilgrims' way churned by the feet and hooves of a thousand mendicants. Traveller's joy was widespread, and there is good reason to believe it was planted by man, or at least that the seeds were scattered by human hand to ensure a plentiful supply for future pilgrimages.

Close contact with cattle and horses led to their handlers suffering periodic outbreaks of that uncomfortable and misnamed fungal skin disease, ringworm, and a poultice of the crushed leaves of old man's beard was thought to be beneficial. Ringworm was the scourge of gypsy peoples, too, and they made up a brew of 3 handfuls of leaves and shoots to half a litre of water, boiled for 10 minutes, then strained and the juice of two lemons added. The acid must have caused the inflamed area to smart unbearably, but the length of time for which this cure held sway before modern preparations took over must say something for its efficacy.

Peppermint
(Mentha x piperita)
Family: LABIATAE

A chance meeting several thousand years ago of two closely related species of mint spawned one of the most popular confectionery flavourings in the world: peppermint. It seems that peppermint is a hybrid of watermint *(Mentha aquatica)* and spearmint *(Mentha spicata)*; the result is a fragrant mixture of the two parents, combining the virtues of both with the typical vigour of a hybrid plant.

Peppermint will seed freely in a herb garden, but usually the seedlings do not breed true to type, so it is best to propagate from root cuttings.

It is a typical mint in that when grown in the right environment it will become invasive, appearing all over the garden as either an annoyance or a delight, depending on your attitude. It doesn't thrive in close proximity to spearmint, and will often vanish from a herb garden altogether in these circumstances. The ruse of planting peppermint in a submerged tub in a herb garden both contains and protects it, ensuring two good crops of leaves and flowers for drying and subsequent use throughout the year.

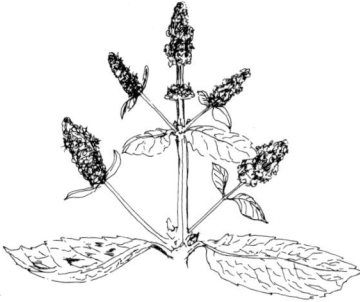

An excellent remedy for an upset stomach is 1 dessertspoonful of peppermint mixed with 1 dessertspoonful of mallow (*Malva sylvestris*) in half a litre of boiling water. Leave for 10 minutes to infuse, then drink while warm. It tastes lovely and needs no sweetening. This will calm heartburn, especially when caused by overeating.

The active ingredients of peppermint are menthol and tannin, both excellent disinfectants. A dressing of peppermint is soothing for cuts and grazes. The leaves are crushed and applied to the graze, where the cooling effect of the menthol helps soothe away any pain.

Essence of peppermint is prepared from flowering plants by a process of steam distillation. This is rather difficult for amateurs and requires expensive specialized equipment, and since essence of oil of peppermint is available from herbal suppliers it's more practical to buy it ready-made.

However, oil of peppermint can be obtained from fresh plants by pounding the leaves, flowers and stems in a mortar. Fill a jar with a tight-fitting lid with this pounded plant, and add olive oil up to the top of the jar. Place on a sunny window-sill for a month, adding fresh pounded plant as the oil breaks down the contents. At the end of a month strain off the oil and press the remaining pulp to expel the last drop. This will keep for a considerable time.

Oil of peppermint relieves wind and stomach cramps. Records going back as far as the thirteenth century cite its use for this purpose all over Europe. Incidentally, it is also the best mint to combine with applemint (*Mentha rotundifolia*) to produce a perfect mint sauce to go with lamb.

Plantain
(Plantago major)
Family: PLANTAGINACEAE

USA: snake weed

Ask any keen gardener his opinion of plantain, and the answer would be less than complimentary, for this low-growing pernicious weed thrives everywhere. Yet in the past, especially in Anglo-Saxon times, plantain was one of the nine sacred herbs, and was called *weybroed*.

The name 'plantain', which is applied to a number of plants of this species, comes from a Latin word for the sole of the foot, and indeed many plantain leaves bear a passing resemblance to the ribbed skin of feet used to walking without the protection of shoes.

Greater plantain is the one that grows most commonly in rockeries and other garden borders, where it soon shades out less robust plants. The thinner-leaved ribwort (*Plantago lanceolata*) is more common on chalk, where it grows freely; indeed, all the common members of this family are free-growing.

Its herbal properties were known to both Greeks and Romans, and were used for treating sores or the bite of a mad dog. More practically, it was applied to stay bleeding, for the leaves do contain an ingredient that suppresses inflammation and reduces bleeding from small wounds.

Greater plantain is still administered in some country districts for nettle stings, and the American Indians used the leaves of this plant as an antidote for snakebite, especially the bite of the rattlesnake. It is still thought to be the best remedy for this, in some tribes. The juice was mixed with salt into a poultice then applied to the bite. The Indians' name for plantain leaf is 'white man's foot', again an allusion to the ribs on the leaves.

When a plant has a multiplicity of names it is often a guide to its degree of usefulness. Plantain falls within this category, with names like 'waybread', 'waybroad', 'greater waybrede', 'slan-lus' (in Scotland) and 'cuckoo's bread'. It's fairly easy to see how these names came about, for members of the plantain family are frequently found growing by paths and roads, often called 'ways' in the past. Pilgrims in Saxon times must have treasured the healing properties of this species, and later on the pil-

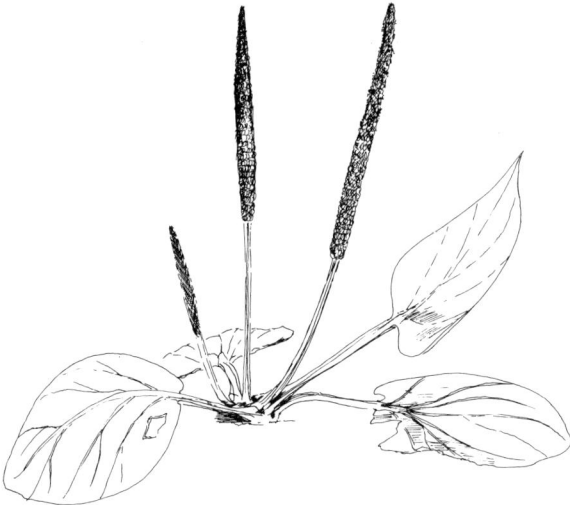

grims of Chaucer's day noted that plantain was good for sprains and ulcers, then both frequent occurrences for travellers.

Culpeper recommended it as a headache remedy, to be mixed with rose oil, and this same compound was used for relieving the pain caused by gout and rheumatism. He also advocated a potion of powdered herbs mixed together with the brine from dried beef. Boiled and clarified, this was considered a wonderful remedy for itchy scalps and other skin infections such as ringworm and shingles.

The ancients were preoccupied with the problems of sores and other skin infections. Their lack of personal hygiene led to chronic infestations of parasites. This, coupled with a general low level of health and nourishment in the population as a whole, meant that an untended sore soon became infected, allowing more serious bacteria to breed and leading to blood poisoning. In consequence, the number of remedies for skin infections were legion.

The whole plant was boiled and the juice drunk after meals for digestive ailments and internal bleeding and as a physic for heavy menstrual flow. It is clear this was a standard use for plantain throughout Europe and the near East. In China the whole plant was cooked and eaten as a vegetable, but the high tannin content gives the leaves and root a bitter taste.

Plantain leaves are an excellent field remedy for minor cuts. If a leaf is bruised and placed on a wound, bleeding will soon stop. Crushed leaves also work wonders on stinging nettle rash, providing, of course, that you apply the leaves immediately after being stung.

Poppy
(Papaver rhoeas)
Family: PAPAVERACEAE

USA: corn poppy, poppy

Poppies have a hard time in our modern countryside. They have been designated weeds by the agricultural community, and as such the full might of the pesticide industry is ranged against them. Yet they still survive in field corners, and splash the landscape like flecks of blood, relieving an otherwise monotonous green.

As food for the soul and medicine for the spirit, poppies, otherwise known as 'corn rose', 'corn poppy' or 'red weed', are well documented and have long been firmly established as a medicinal herb. Another of the country names is 'headache', which came about because the flower heads were used in an infusion to relieve headache symptoms.

The history of poppies goes back many thousands of years to the ancient Egyptians. They festooned the tombs of their kings and dignitaries with garlands of poppy flowers. The dry atmosphere of the Valley of the Kings preserved the

poppy seeds because they were said to be good for keeping intestinal movements regular. In the words of Dioscorides, 'It doth soften the belly gently.'

Poppy seeds as a culinary ingredient are still popular to this day, with poppy-seeded bread and rolls. However, during the Middle Ages poppies were more often pressed into service for treating pleurisy and other chest infections. The flowers were dried and crushed and infused in hot water, and again we use them similarly today.

Almost all preparations made with the flowers, that is, the petals themselves, should be treated in a special way in order to ensure that the potency is not lost in the drying process. Poppy petals are as delicate as tissue paper and should be dried quickly in order not to lose their colour. They should be handled with extreme care whilst fresh, for if crushed they will dry black and useless. An airing cupboard is the perfect place; when they are dry crush them and store in dark-glass bottles away from damp and light.

Poppies are known to have a slightly narcotic effect, but it is not harmful, in fact it has been recommended for relieving angina and asthma (though these two illnesses are far too serious to treat yourself without expert guidance). However, they can be very effective in cases of colic, where the herb's soothing properties can calm stomach spasms. Poppy also

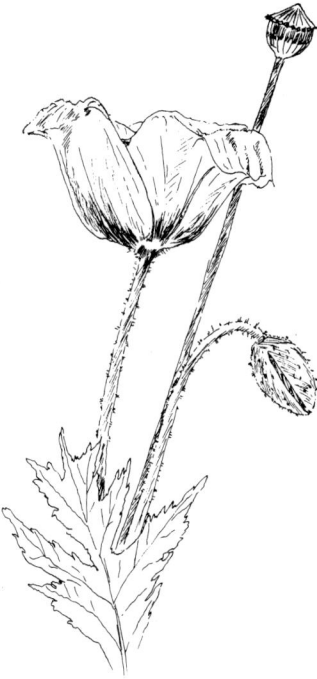

flowers in such perfection that they were easily recognizable. It is quite clear that poppies must have bloomed in an Egypt rather different in climate from the arid landscape of today.

The Pharoahs not only decorated their tombs with poppy flowers, they used them for medicinal purposes and the seeds as decoration on cakes and sweetmeats, as did the Romans, who inherited the Egyptians' taste for luxury and the good things in life. The Romans had, in fact, a profound interest in the lifestyle of the Egyptians, and were also keen on

has the power to raise a person's temperature slightly to promote perspiration.

The common poppy and opium poppy (*Papaver somniferum*) belong to the same family, although the active ingredients present in the common variety are far weaker. Opium poppies grow in the hot climate of the East and the Indian sub-continent.

Nevertheless, the common poppy has been associated with its potent cousin by family connection, and was used as a mild sleeping draught for past generations of infants – not that this is any recommendation, for in Hogarth's time mothers used to give their babies neat gin to still their cries!

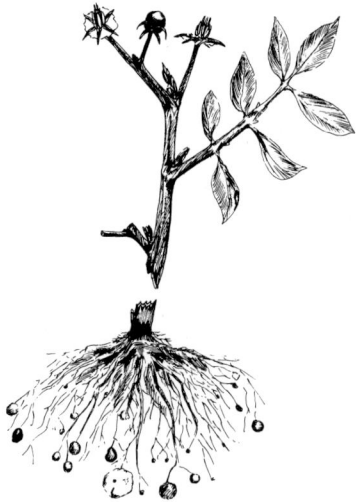

Potato

(Solanum tuberosum)
Family: SOLANACEAE

It would be hard to imagine life without the humble potato. Since its introduction from the New World in the sixteenth century it has become a staple food. Perhaps the potato famines that occurred in Ireland helped influence the many Irish families who left their Emerald Isle for a new life in America.

The potato, which has spawned a multi-million-pound fast-food industry, was once looked upon with dread, for it was thought to cause scurvy, and it belongs to the genus solanum which has among its relatives belladonna and the henbanes,

to name just a few used by poisoners down the centuries.

This fear of potatoes has some basis in fact, because the fruit – the berry-like potato apples that follow the flower – have a rather unpleasant effect if you eat them, and potato tubers, if allowed to go green after exposure to sunlight, acquire a high content of oxalic acid. Cooked potato should never be stored in unrefrigerated conditions, for it is a perfect medium for noxious bacteria.

Notwithstanding these facts, the potato has become king among staple foods in the West, and there are about 1,600 different varieties.

In essence a tropical plant, it has been adapted by time and plant breeders to our climate, but ideally it would prefer equal days and nights, such as you would find near the equator. In its natural habitat it makes far fewer and smaller root tubers, and the toxicity of the fruit would deter all but the hungriest grazer.

Apart from their culinary value, potato tubers, which we have developed to a larger size, are used for a variety of country medicines. Because they contain vitamin C just below the skin they were used to relieve and prevent the very disease they were thought to cause – the dreaded deficiency disease of scurvy, particularly prevalent in seamen and also in the urban population of the eighteenth century. Even in these enlightened times when fresh fruit is available all year round, potatoes provide much of the vitamin C in our average diet.

This vitamin is thought to have the power to relieve and shorten some effects of the common cold, and though there is very little scientific positive proof that it can do this many people swear by massive doses of vitamin C. Vitamin C does seem to have certain powers when applied to the skin to relieve some skin infections. It allows skin to heal more rapidly, and possibly this was why raw grated potato was recommended as a cold poultice for mild skin infections and boils.

The high vitamin and mineral content could also account for raw potato juice being prescribed as a herbal remedy for ulcers. When taken in this way it is usual to make a cocktail of potato juice, carrot juice and honey to modify the taste. This cocktail was often recommended as a general tonic, and there can be little doubt that the minerals and vitamins contained in it would be very beneficial to health – providing, of course, that it is absolutely fresh.

Boiled floury potatoes mashed to a creamy consistency with a little milk and a few drops of glycerin and rose water can be applied to soften and whiten hands and skin. Slices of raw potato placed on the eyelids are supposed to reduce wrinkling, and cuts that are slow to heal will sometimes respond to raw potato slices applied as a dressing, as will blind boils and other painful swellings. Ensure any potatoes used are thoroughly cleaned.

Clearly, the potato is not just a constituent of the well-known, well-loved British favourite of fish and chips!

Quince

(Cydonia oblonga)
Family: ROSACEAE

Cottage gardens in the south of England once supported large numbers of shrubby quince trees. Now there are relatively few of the original stock remaining. They have the appearance of a small misshapen apple tree, with similar leaves but larger and rather more downy on the underside.

Quince blossom is extremely attractive and rose-like, as befits a

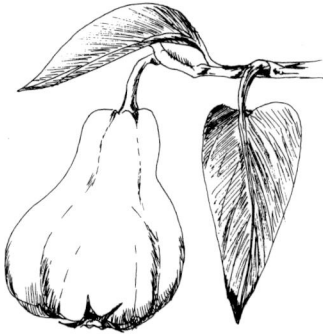

member of the family *rosaceae*, but it also has the lovely qualities of apple blossom, with a sweet if rather fleeting scent. After the blossom comes the fruit, which in medicinal terms is the most important part of the tree.

Quince is not native to Britain, being thought to originate from the Mediterranean, and consequently the fruit is late in ripening. Even when ripe, the pear-shaped fruits with their fluted surface are coarse-textured and difficult to eat. They can become more palatable when affected by frost, as the fibres are broken down somewhat.

Few culinary recipes incorporate quince fruit, other than as an ingredient in pies and jellies. Quince jelly was a favourite food for invalids in the late Victorian era.

Quince seeds are found in a mass at the core of the fruit, and contain a mucilin in their coat. They are not palatable, and overdose is rare. Mucilage extracted from the seed coat by soaking seeds in boiling water for about 10 minutes looks like egg white. This extract can be used to soothe and calm both stomach and digestive system after diarrhoea, and although it has been used in the past as a mild laxative, the mucilage generally has a beneficial effect on disorders of the lower bowel. It can also be dissolved in warm water to make a gargle and a mouthwash, and Culpeper recommended mucilage of quince as a lotion for sore breasts.

In Spain the inner peel is known for its healing properties and is considered a good hair tonic. The peel of 3 quinces is boiled in half a litre of water for ten minutes, then left to cool. This same recipe was also employed in certain countries as a treatment for venereal disease.

Raspberry
(Rubus idaeus)
Family: ROSACEAE

Deep red raspberries are the most delicious of wild fruit, though it's difficult to think of them as wild, for there are very few native raspberry plants in our modern countryside.

They have been affected by the cultivation of high-yielding strains, and many plants growing at the woodland's edge or around the margins of common land owe their propagation, not to nature, but to kitchen gardeners who have dumped their prunings there along with other refuse, to the detriment of countryside flora. The cuttings

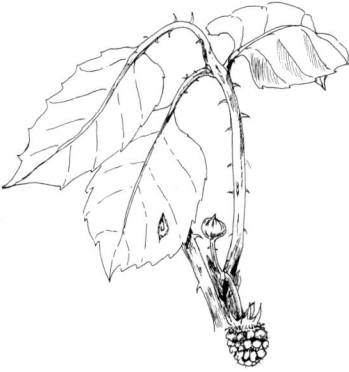

that take root and fruit have little of the natural hardiness of true wild plants and are susceptible to virus infections which render them less suitable for medicinal purposes. However, if you have a source of uncontaminated raspberries you may consider yourself fortunate.

In the days when bears roamed the Chiltern Hills and had their lairs in beechwoods, gathering raspberries was a chancy business, for they seem to be the favourite fruit of bears. In Russia and northern Europe, where European brown bears still live, you can get quite close to these animals if you are brave enough, so intent are they feasting on the luscious fruit.

Raspberries were firm favourites with the Romanies as a general tonic, and raspberry flower tea or a similar infusion made with leaves and young shoots is an excellent treatment for influenza. Herbalists sell dried raspberry leaves and flowers, but they are common enough in gardens to be used fresh.

Tea made from raspberry leaves was used by women during pregnancy as a tonic for the uterus to ensure fewer complications in labour, and its astringent qualities were said to be good for relieving morning sickness and also for digestive ailments in infants.

A lotion of infused leaves is supposed to be good for toning up skin, but before applying any herbal preparations externally, especially a very active one like raspberry, it's best to check for allergic reaction on a small area of skin, preferably on the forearm. If there is any irritation after 10 minutes, don't use it.

Raspberries make a lovely cordial. Heat about 1 kilogram of fruit in a stainless steel saucepan and add a little honey to taste. When the fruit is soft squeeze through a muslin bag or pulp in a liquidizer, then leave to cool. An expectant mother could do worse than to drink this cordial or raspberry leaf tea throughout her pregnancy, and eat ripe raspberries in season, though perhaps without cream and sugar.

Rhubarb
(Rheum officinale, Rheum palmatum)
Family: POLYGONACEAE

We do not normally think of rhubarb as a medicinal plant, yet the Chinese set great store by its res-

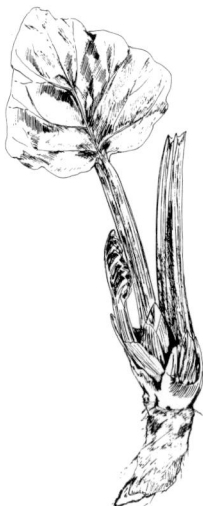

torative principles and used it widely in many differing remedies. In Britain it is best known as a main ingredient in tarts, pies, crumbles or *compotes*, usually accompanied by custard.

The long reddish mottled stems are a decalcifying agent, rich in acid, and in Victorian times old iron kettles were cleared of lime-scale by the expedient of boiling a handful of chopped rhubarb stems in the kettle – this method is just as valid today. However, the kettle must be treated several times and all the scale removed, or a strong rhubarb flavour will linger in the remaining lime deposit.

The acid content in the stems is one reason why rhubarb wine can be less than successful. Yeast organisms find the acidity level in the juice much too high and often

refuse to propagate, fooling wine-makers into thinking that the ferment is sticking because of lack of sweetness. Consequently they add more sugar to the must, which sometimes starts a dull ferment that eventually peters out because of excess acid, and leaves the wine-maker with a brew too sweet for anyone's taste-buds.

To reduce acidity add precipitated chalk, and continue adding it until the mixture is just slightly acid on a proprietory indicator. It will then ferment freely and produce a better end result.

Rhubarb wine is recognized as good for the digestion if taken in moderation, and the fruity stem itself has long been used for treating bowel disorders. It was made much of between the wars as a laxative, and a generation of children born at that time came to loathe the sight of it.

To prepare a mild tonic, the root first has to be gathered and dried. This can be a long process, for it has to be taken from plants that are over five years old, and they are usually well entrenched and require considerable effort to remove them. When mature they can be as thick as a man's arm and more than $\frac{1}{2}$m long, and the reddish hard bark-like covering has to be scraped away to reveal the ivory-white or yellow flesh. Cut the root into sugar-cube sized pieces and dry in an airing cupboard on a netted frame. It is resistant to drying and often takes a month to become completely dessicated.

Infuse 10g of crushed root for 10 minutes in 1 litre of boiling water to produce a mildly laxative tonic drink, or the stems can be eaten raw with a little honey to reduce sharpness. This provides fibre and a mild purgative action that will not normally cause colic; and the stewed fruit stems prepared as a dessert also give a general beneficial effect.

A word of warning, though, about rhubarb leaves. They contain poisonous oxalic acid, which can be fatal in relatively small doses and will certainly cause intense stomach irritation. However, organic gardeners put this toxic property to good effect as a weedkiller; it is especially powerful in dealing with creeping grasses such as couch grass and on other weeds with roots near the surface. The poison seems to reduce the plant's ability to gather nutrients and creates an environment that few plants can tolerate.

The leaves should be laid over a weedy area and allowed to stay there, if necessary covering with black polythene to exclude all light. The combination of leaf acid and lack of ultra-violet so inhibits the weeds that they will go elsewhere or just give up the ghost altogether. The advantage of this form of treatment is that the soil soon becomes clear of any rhubarb acid and is not polluted, whereas synthetic chemicals often persist in the soil, to be taken up by vegetables or other edible plants.

Rue, common
(Ruta graveolens)
Family: RUTACEAE

One has only to look at rue to see its Mediterranean origins. The hard grey leaves are specially designed to resist drought, and the plant is most at home on dry stony ground with hot sun and not much rainfall.

Yet it is to be found growing vigorously in herb gardens all over Britain. The woody stems spread from a central base like an ornamental shrub which can reach heights of up to 1m.

Rue is surrounded by legend. It was well known and documented by the Greeks, who were recipients of medical cultures from previous civilizations. Dioscorides recommended it as a remedy for snakebite because legend had it that weasels ate the bitter-tasting leaves before battling with poisonous snakes.

It seems likely that this legend was borrowed from further east than Greece. It could well have originated from travellers on the silk routes as they journeyed across Asia, particularly India where the mongoose, a weasel-like animal, regularly fought with snakes without being bitten and was therefore thought to have the power to resist snakebite through recourse to an antidote. One can easily imagine how the story was embellished, especially if the listeners were more familiar with weasels than with the mongoose.

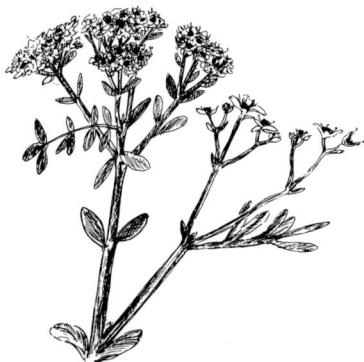

Similar embellishments of the powers of other plants probably came about in much the same way. That there are few poisonous snakes in Europe and even fewer in the British Isles, where this legend was also propagated by Gerard, was always a well-known fact, yet there are very many remedies for snakebite in herbals of the Middle Ages.

In the East rue is grown for its magical power to keep households from evil. It is said to be the only plant blessed by the prophet Mohammed. Its magical powers were established between the fourteenth and seventeenth centuries, when as well as being adopted in church celebrations of mass it was also widely recognized as an ingredient in exorcism rituals.

It was considered an excellent herb for strewing, especially where there were contagious ills and fleas. The law courts were liberally strewn with branches and twigs of rue to protect the Officers of the Court from gaol fever, and from such insect visitors as prisoners brought into the dock with them from their foul cells.

Medicinally, rue contains a compound called rutocide, which is toxic in large quantities and was used in the past to procure abortions by causing contraction of the womb and the onset of menstrual bleeding. Poor diet and heavy work for peasants on the one hand and overfed dissolute landed gentry on the other frequently led to menstrual disorders for both classes, and rue was employed by all to restore the normal cycle.

It is also known as a culinary herb, although the pungent taste is not generally popular, but it is suitable as an appetizer when administered in small doses. Small doses are also helpful to ease colic and tone up the system. However, serious side-effects can arise if too much is taken, with symptoms similar to drunkenness and frenzy.

Dried flowers of rue were applied as a lotion for poor sight, and dried powdered plant can be mixed with a little distilled water as a skin treatment for minor inflammation, but fresh leaves should be applied as an emergency dressing for cuts.

Sage
(Salvia officinalis)
Family: LABIATAE

Many plants contain medicinal properties that are used by the

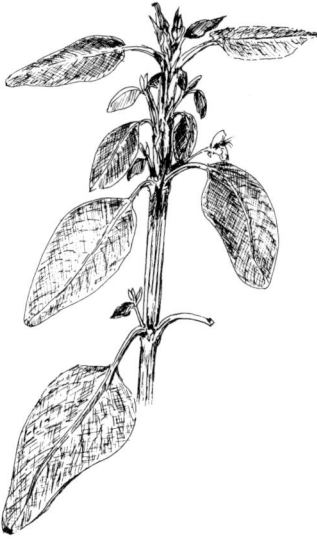

plants themselves as a means of protection, especially those that grow in hot or sub-tropical lands.

For centuries flocks of sheep and goats have grazed the goodness out of the soil until the only plants left are those that can protect themselves with spines or tough unpalatable leaves or toxins, causing animals that venture to eat them to become ill and to learn not to try it again. In consequence, plants like sage flourish in many countries.

Although we grow it for culinary purposes, sage has an illustrious history as a medicinal plant.

Ancient Egyptians revered it as both giver and saver of life, and regarded it as a treatment for plague, while Ancient Greeks thought it could render man immortal. This does overstate its power somewhat, but the Romans prized sage to such a degree that harvesting the blue-green leaves was conducted as a ceremony rather than an ordinary gardening event.

Indeed, it was gathered with bronze or silver tools, iron not being considered good enough, and the gatherers had to be clean, dressed in white tunics, and barefoot. Prior to harvesting gatherers would offer sacrifices of food and wine to the gods.

However, there are less pleasant aspects of this paragon of herbs. Taken in excess, an infusion of sage can be harmful in that it promotes an excessive flow of blood to the gut and there could be possible effects on the central nervous system. Fortunately, it is not a herb normally used in large doses.

The Romans prescribed sage for childless couples who fervently wished to conceive. The couple remained apart for four days drinking sage juice, then enjoyed a second honeymoon. It was said to be unfailing in its effect.

The Romans were not the only ones to use sage for this purpose. Egyptians considered it an excellent fertility drug and much sage juice was drunk after the great plagues of Egypt. The results must have been satisfactory, for sage continued to be recommended throughout the ages.

Its Latin name is full of meaning, salvia being derived from the Latin *salvare*, to save or to cure, and in the Middle Ages sage was employed by herbalists as a last resort. Infant mortality was rampant, and a tea made from sage leaves was given to very sick children when all else had failed and there was nothing to lose. A spoonful every 5 minutes was the prescribed amount.

There could well be a genuine reason why sage tea was of value, for the killer diseases of infanthood were usually intestinal ailments where a child could lose vast quantities of body fluids with no way of recovering them because of loss of appetite. The water of those days was less than helpful to a damaged digestive system, as it was frequently polluted.

Sage has an antiseptic property that would have destroyed any germs left after the water had been heated to prepare a medicine. It is also a sedative, and would probably have had a quietening effect on the digestion so that the child would be more relaxed and less inclined to vomiting and diarrhoea. Lastly, the herb has the power to reduce temperature.

But it could be that, apart from these healing properties, the frequent quantities of sterile water making up an infusion would be replacing liquid lost by the child, and therefore reducing dehydration and the possibility of kidney failure.

St John's wort
(Hypericum perforatum)
Family: GUTTIFERAE

St John's wort is well proven in its efficacy. Greeks, Romans and many other European warriors, including the Crusaders, took this plant to war with them to act as a styptic for bleeding and as a salve to heal wounds and burns.

The name 'St John's wort' is thought to have come about because the stems yield a red pigment likened to the blood of John the Baptist. This red coloration, known as hypericum red (hypericine) was recommended as an infusion in small doses to relieve pain.

St John's wort's fame goes far beyond its ability to heal wounds. It is credited with the power to keep houses safe from evil spirits, and in the past those unfortunate souls who suffered mental illness or epilepsy or delusions were made to sniff the juice to drive out the evil spirits supposedly detected in them.

Witchcraft apart, the power of this plant to relieve inflammation and heal wounds and scalds is real enough. Taken internally, it was prescribed for a variety of ills, from upsets of the bile duct to gastric disorders of many sorts and also to treat irregular and painful periods. A tea was made with 2 tablespoons of dried plant in cold water. This was brought slowly to the boil, removed from the heat and allowed

After sun and time have done their work you will be left with an amber-coloured oil smelling pleasantly spicy. Filter to reduce sediment, and bottle for future use.

This oil is especially effective for cracked dry skin, caused by chapping in cold weather or solvents and detergents.

Shepherd's purse
(Capsella bursa-pastoris)
Family: CRUCIFERAE

Shepherd's purse is a rather humble weed, but few other plants possess such healing powers.

In the Middle Ages, shepherd's purse was used to stem bleeding caused by cuts from edged tools and weapons, and in some areas of Britain it is known as St James's wort, a herb blessed by the church.

In gypsy encampments it was applied in conjunction with spider's webs to stop bleeding. The method adopted was to make a strong infusion, pour it into the wound, then plug the open area with webs. The logic of using webs in this way is well founded, for as blood clots naturally it forms a network of fibrins to bind the clot firmly. Spider's web is an artificial fibrin which forms a good trap for solids in the wound.

The name 'shepherd's purse' doesn't refer to any use made of this herb by shepherds, although many of them were skilled in herbal remedies and doctored their

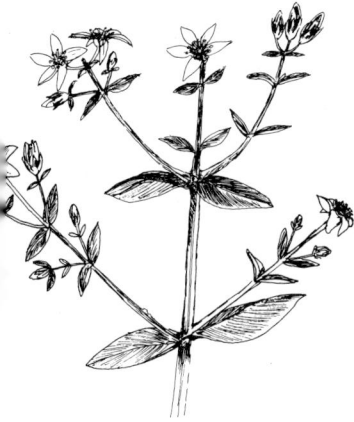

to stand until cool. A cupful was then taken 3 times a day.

However, the advisability of taking St John's wort as an internal medicine is now in doubt. In some cases, extreme sensitivity to light can result, indicating that in large doses the plant's constituent hypericine may have an adverse effect on the central nervous system, although the dose would have to be very high. This effect was first noticed in animals grazing on the plant in summer.

Nevertheless, oil of St John's wort is a valuable salve for cuts and grazes, bruises and scalds, where its action can be marked. To prepare an oil, fill a glass jar (kilner jars are best) with flowering heads, top up the jar with olive oil and seal. Place the jar in the sun for four weeks and shake daily to ensure the oil penetrates the plant thoroughly. As the contents settle, put more fresh plant in.

own sheep even after modern medicines and veterinary practice came into being. The name comes from the heart-shaped seed capsules, which resemble the leather pouches carried by shepherds on their belts. It was also called 'mother's heart'.

It is very common indeed, and a member of the cabbage family, the same botanical group as honesty and wallflowers. The leaves are similar in shape to deeply cut dark-green dandelion leaves, and the seeds and flowers are carried on a spire of stems that can rise to over 30cm high in favoured sunny positions. Often this plant will take over rubble and newly turned ground, as it is able to thrive on poor soil. The flowers are so small as to be insignificant, the whitish petals soon dropping after fertilization.

Because it is so common it's best to use shepherd's purse fresh, for it is one of those herbs that tends to lose some of its properties when dried. However, it will freeze well and should be stored in an airtight container to avoid dessication.

As an infusion to reduce the effects of heavy, painful menstrual bleeding, soak a handful of fresh plant in 1 litre of boiling water for 20 minutes to produce the correct level of active ingredients. Strain, and drink a cupful before meals.

French herbals recommend that an infusion should be taken 24 hours before the onset of menstruation to lessen the severity of symptoms.

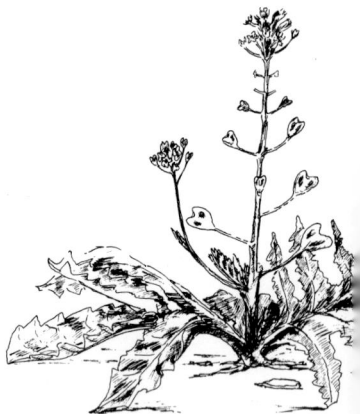

As a general tonic this plant has many benefits, and a tea made from the same proportions as given above tones up a sluggish system and promotes a feeling of well-being. You will have to take a cup of this tea every day for 3 or 4 weeks before you will notice its good effects.

Tea made from shepherd's purse can have an unpleasant flavour, but the plant can be made more acceptable if prepared in a wine. To do this, soak 90g of chopped shepherd's purse in half a litre of wine for 8 days, then strain. One small wine glass 3 times a day is the prescribed dose.

Lastly, the plant has acquired a reputation for stopping nose-bleeds. Prepare a strong infusion of 2 handfuls of fresh herbs to 1 litre of boiling water, cool, and sniff up the nose or apply on a plug of clean lint.

Silver birch

(Betula pendula)

Family: BETULACEAE

Few trees are better endowed with real or imaginary healing powers than the beautiful and stately birch. 'Lady of the forest' and 'silver birch' are two of the many names by which this tree is known in Europe and Asia.

A short-lived tree in woodland terms, it rarely survives longer than ninety years, but its fast-growing qualities helped to heal our island landscape after the devastation of the last ice age.

When the ice retreated it left land as bleak as if an atomic bomb had been dropped; no living things survived in the sterile soil, and even the worms had died of intense cold and the staggering weight of the ice. To gain some idea of the weight of glaciers that stretched from the Arctic to what is now London and beyond, it is necessary to realize that they pressed the earth's crust downward so much that when the ice melted the land surface rose many feet, and indeed it is still recovering and rising slightly.

Into this sterile scene came the first spores of mosses and lichens, drifting on cold winds that swept unhindered from all points of the compass. Gradually these plants tamed the scratched rock and powdery silt in the valleys, providing a seed bed for heather and ling, but there were still no plants of any height. The seeds of birch, perhaps

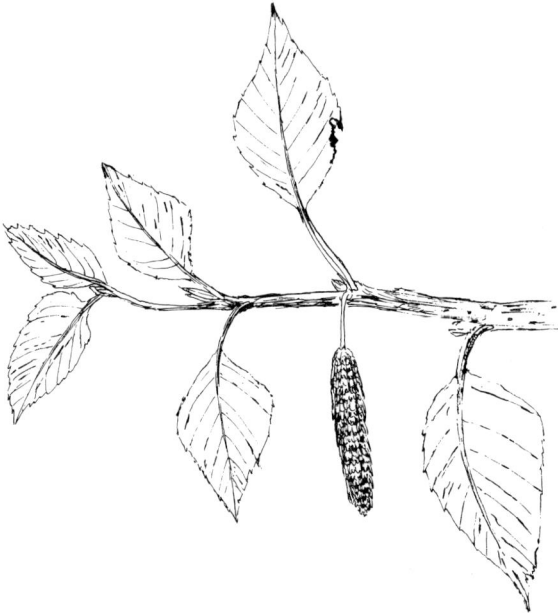

carried into the area by the pelts of reindeer, mammoth and woolly rhino, were the first to find a roothold. They tucked their roots into crevices and began to colonize valleys where they could survive the bitter winter winds. As the climate improved, so the birch forests spread to cover and heal the land. The short lifespan of birch and its soft wood which rotted readily meant that within a few thousand years there was enough topsoil and leaf mould for other less tough trees to gain rootholds in the forests.

Our primitive ancestors drifted back into these islands and found that birch was a useful antiseptic. In spring a birch tree pushes up sap into its trunk with such power that if a hole is bored in the tree with an auger and a straw inserted, the sap will flow freely. In Scandinavia birch is milked in this way; two weeks is usually the longest length of time allowed before the small hole is plugged with a clean wooden peg. Great care must then be taken to sterilize the wound, or moulds will enter the tree and kill it.

'Birch water' is the name by which the sap is known after it has been gathered, and it has long been used as a remedy for kidney infections. In Napoleon's campaigns the French surgeon general was so impressed by the efficacy of birch water that he called it a universal panacea for peasant and gentry alike, which would cure infections of the skin, was valuable as a remedy for rheumatism and was wonderful 'for relieving the after-effects of gout and blockages of the bladder'.

Two hundred years before the surgeon general made his pronouncement, the Spanish physician Matthiolus had said that 'the water which cometh out of the birch tree was wondrous for breaking the stones in kidneys or gall bladder'. This must have been an ailment which frequently afflicted our forefathers, for in all the herbals from many countries there are references to such medicines.

The method of treatment was to lay the patient on a bed of birch leaves covered over with more birch leaves and then a blanket, so that the body heat built up. The closeness of the birch leaves was thought soothing, and this treatment, together with a glass of birch water, was said to give long-lasting relief from pain.

Silverweed
(Potentilla anserina)
Family: ROSACEAE

Silverweed belongs to a herbal genus known generally as potentilla. Even the name sounds effective, and there are three species common enough to be used medicinally, the most common being silverweed itself. It thrives alongside paths and waste places, especially on chalk soil, and it has been valued since pre-Roman times.

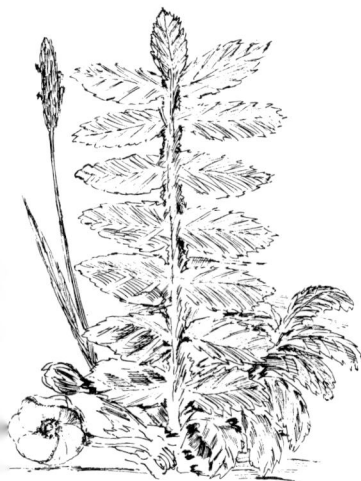

During times of famine women from the nomadic tribes of Britain would dig the roots for food. They make a tough morsel, but are rich in minerals and some vitamins, and were no doubt welcome enough to keep body and soul together.

Loss of many of our wild places and reduction in available uncultivated land has meant that silverweed is not as common as it once was, and chemical manufacturers have provided an armoury of poisons with which to eradicate it from the garden. However, to destroy it is to lose a remedy for many minor ailments, as both leaves and flowers are rich in tannin.

The silver foliage and bright delicate golden flowers should make it a favourite with herb gardeners. It can be invasive, but if controlled by pulling up the smaller plants it will repay your trouble.

Along with other members of the family it is famous as a remedy for the painful and embarrassing condition of bleeding piles. A medicine for this condition, also recommended for treating cystitis, can be prepared by soaking 30g of dried leaves and flowers in 1 litre of cold water for an hour. Bring this mixture to the boil and simmer for 10 minutes, then cool and strain off into a clean glass container. One cupful before meals 3 times a day should have a beneficial effect.

As with most herbal medicines, it is essential to prepare a fresh mixture as and when required. Any mixture not used should be thrown away; do not store it for more than a day or two. All the potentillas should be dried quickly in the sun to avoid moulds growing and destroying their potency, and they should be stored in dark bottles, tightly stoppered.

Silverweed has two other useful herbal relatives, cinquefoil (*Potentilla reptans*) and tormentil (*Potentilla erecta*).

Cinquefoil is the plant the Ancient Egyptians used to allay the symptoms of malaria, a very common illness in that country so dependent on the riverside habitat of the Nile where mosquitoes flourish. It is still used to reduce fevers and stomach cramps. A member of the family rosaceae, it can be confused with wild strawberry, to which it is related. The reddish stems will spread like strawberry runners and cover large areas of grassland, so if you grow it for medicinal purposes keep it in a pot or in a small tub and use the runners as they flower.

The last of the three is tormentil, and this is the most potent. An infusion of flowers and leaves (30g to 1 litre of water – prepared as for silverweed) is good for colic and diarrhoea and is frequently prescribed by herbalists as a most effective treatment for cystitis. It has also been prescribed for hay fever and bronchial trouble, and for heavy periods. Externally it is an excellent treatment for eczema and dry itching skin and in the past was made into a dressing for ulcers.

Chewing a piece of root will relieve gum boils, and a brew of leaves and flowers is a valuable gargle for sore throats. Tormentil root can also be made into a very pleasant effective tonic wine by crushing 60g of fresh root and adding 1 litre of white wine. Leave for about a week before straining. The dose is 1 small wineglassful per day.

A tincture of the root, which has the same tonic properties, is prepared by soaking 50g of dried ground root in a quarter of a litre of vodka or some other clear spirit like schnapps for 30 days. This should be strained and pressed through a fine cloth, and the resulting liquid taken diluted in water or alternatively a few drops on a lump of sugar. The advantage of tinctures is that they last a long time, as alcohol ensures preservation.

Just a word of warning, though.

Never prepare infusions of acrid plants (those high in tannin content) in steel or iron vessels, as the pots and pans will discolour and the brew will take on a metallic taste.

Soapwort
(Saponaria officinalis)
Family: CARYOPHYLLACEAE

USA: bouncing Bet, fuller's herb, hedge pink, old man's pink, soapwort, wild sweet-william

Over the past few years there has been considerable discussion as to the authenticity of that famous religious relic, the Turin Shroud. It keeps its secret for the moment, but it is only a matter of time before chemical analysis will reveal whether the marks are those of a crucified body or the work of an extremely clever forger. The romantic in me hopes that scientists will remain confounded and the legend sustained, for there is no way of knowing for certain if the image is that of Jesus of Nazareth.

Investigations into the substance of the Shroud have revealed various intensely interesting facts about life and fabrics in the early centuries of the past millennium. It appears that the linen was woven, rather like modern twill, from flax fibres and exposed to pollen from plants that grow in the Middle East, but it was because the shroud was washed with common soapwort that it is still with us.

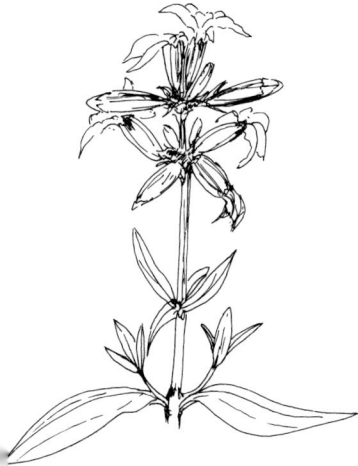

Soapwort, which once inhabited many damp ditches and flowery meadows, was the plant our ancestors used to get their washing whiter-than-white, and it is a very effective fungicide, a major factor in preserving cloth in such good order for so many centuries. The root is the part from which the soapy extract is expressed, although the leaves are also useful in soap-making.

This plant has a host of country names; 'soaproot', 'crow soap', 'crowther soap', 'latherwort', and there's a direct allusion to the past industry of wool treatment in one of its other names, 'fuller's herb'. It is also called bouncing betty, perhaps referring to washerwomen who may have enjoyed the luxury of soft hands using this natural product.

The Greeks were familiar with its properties as a detergent and as a medicine, and Gerard said that 'it scoureth almost as good as soap'. It was widely employed to keep the surface of wooden eating bowls clean and wholesome. This was due as much to its power to destroy bacteria as to its ability to remove grease and stains.

Soapwort was used to treat rather severe skin ailments and possibly even leprosy, which was not uncommon in the Middle Ages. However, it was more widely used for the treatment of venereal disease. Massive doses were prescribed ($\frac{1}{2}$ oz of juice to be taken daily) and it's likely that sufferers could well have been hastened off this mortal coil, for the plant contains a substance (saponin glycoside) which can cause violent gastro-enteritis followed by depression of the function of the central nervous system.

Less harmful was the practice of 'snuffing' soapwort. It caused violent sneezing, which was thought to relieve illness.

It was widely exploited well into the nineteenth century for liver infections and to relieve rheumatic symptoms. The plant can still be purchased from reputable herbalists for treating skin ailments, but its toxic qualities have caused it to fall from favour as a medicine.

However, its soapy character is still much in demand. Tapestries and medieval wall hangings that are being restored and conserved in our museums and research institutes do not as a rule take kindly to modern detergents, but respond well to treatment with an extract of soapwort, just as the Turin Shroud has done.

Spearmint
(Mentha spicata)
Family: LABIATAE

The main ingredient of spearmint, one of the parents of peppermint hybrids, is a volatile element known as carvone, the same compound as is extracted from caraway seeds. It is this that gives spearmint its characteristic scent.

Spearmint is best known for flavouring confectionery, especially chewing gum, and toothpaste. The connection between dental care and spearmint goes back a long way; there are records in Greek and Roman herbal writings of coarse spearmint leaves being employed as a rub for keeping teeth clean and the breath sweet.

The smell of spearmint is less pleasant when expressed from the fresh plant than when prepared as an oil by the same method as that employed for peppermint or as an infusion of dried plant. Spearmint as a scent was well known to Greeks and Romans, who added it to their bath water where its property of stimulating the skin and acting as a mild antiseptic was invaluable after the heat of the day.

Medicinally, it has been administered to ease stomach cramps and was thought suitable as a remedy for jaundice. There are several references in modern herbals to its use for liver ailments, though there is little evidence as to the efficacy of this treatment.

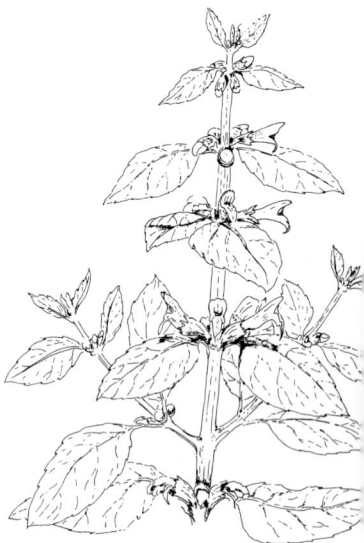

It is a general calming agent for the stomach and may have an effect on bile secretion. It was recommended by Culpeper as a cure for hiccoughs, vomiting and, if our interpretation of his words is correct, as a type of aphrodisiac, for he says that it stirs up venery or bodily lust. As it is also recommended to suppress lactation, ease pains in the ears and stay bleeding, it would seem that by the sixteenth century spearmint had gathered a considerable reputation as a healing plant.

Moreover, despite all the conjecture, spearmint is an excellent herb for stomach upsets and can form a very effective emergency toothpaste and mouthwash for sore gums.

Sphagnum moss
(Sphagnum cymbifolium)
Family: MUSCI

This was very likely the first really green plant to return to England and the northern United States as ice sheets retreated after the last ice age. The passage of millions of tons of crushing ice milled rocks to a gravelly paste as it flowed across the landscape, leaving behind depressions in the land which filled with silt and water. Spores, borne on the wind, colonized the virgin rocks with a luxuriant carpet of sphagnum moss, like a green bandage allowing the land to heal its scars beneath a protecting layer.

The analogy with a bandage is used advisedly, for there is little doubt that hunter-gatherer tribes of Stone Age wanderers valued moss for bandaging their cuts and grazes as they followed herds of reindeer and mammoth on their long migrations. From that time until the present day, sphagnum moss has served mankind in a hundred different ways.

The decomposition of sphagnum moss in a bog is carried on without oxygen and may take many thousands of years to complete. The best garden peat is gathered from areas where sphagnum moss grew most abundantly.

Barber-surgeons of the Middle Ages applied moss as a bandage to heal infected wounds, for when dry it has the power to absorb many times it own weight in water. During the First World War the horrors of trench warfare were almost inconceivable, with all manner of wounds sustained and treated by the most inadequate and primitive methods, often in field

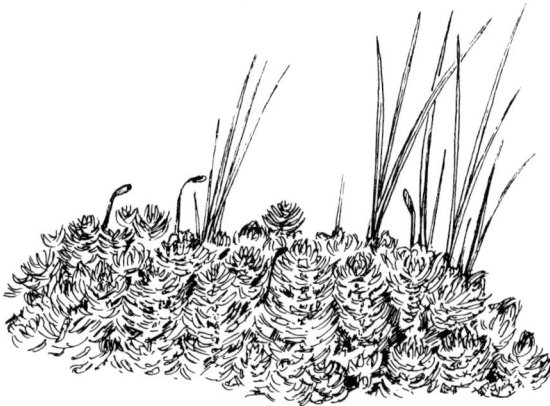

conditions by untried orderlies. Gas gangrene was common, and many men died through lack of medicaments from wounds which would have healed with the help of modern powerful antibiotics, but there are people alive to this day who owe their lives to the application of dried sphagnum moss to their festering wounds.

Sometimes sphagnum moss was employed in conjunction with garlic. Garlic has its own antibiotic action which is enhanced by antibiotic properties in the moss and the ability of this moss to draw moisture away from an affected area, so reducing saturation of tissues. This allowed wounds to begin the process of healing, even where the body's own defence mechanism had been weakened. In spite of the appalling conditions of the trenches, the cold and the poor diet, some wounded men responded.

American Indians also applied sphagnum moss as a wound dressing and to stem bleeding, and again wild garlic was used in conjunction with the moss.

Sphagnum moss often grows in conditions of relative sterility. The high acid content of the ground water into which its roots search is a hostile environment for many harmful organisms, but even so, should you consider employing sphagnum moss as a wound dressing, sterilize it by boiling it before drying.

A moss bandage would rarely have been wasted, for there is a long history of Irish horse doctors whose treatments included bandages for their charges, especially for those sores caused by unfeeling owners who allowed a chafing harness to rub needlessly.

Sunflower
(Helianthus annuus)
Family: COMPOSITAE

The Aztecs venerated sunflowers, and it is easy to see why. Tall and stately, the flowers closely resemble the sun they worshipped, and the plant itself rewarded them in godlike fashion with food, oil and a medicine all in one package.

Even the inside part of the stem saved life. It is exceptionally light, and in the Americas of the eighteenth century it was made into life-preserving buoyancy aids similar to the lifebuoys that rescuers throw to people in difficulty in the water. A very necessary form of safety equipment it must have been, for sailors in those days were often poor swimmers.

The majority of sunflowers are cultivated in Russia, Spain and North America. Sunflower is a traditional crop of the East, where the seeds are used to feed animals, but this is a rather wasteful use of the oil-rich seeds, for they have a very high protein content, in some cases as high as 50%, which is extremely easy to assimilate.

However, it is the actual sunflower oil that has caused so much

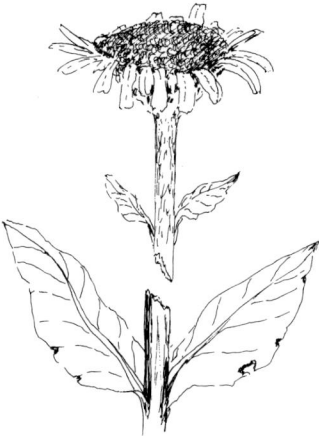

interest over the past few years. When expressed from the seeds and purified, it is extremely low in those fatty substances thought to contribute to coronary heart disease. The palatable oil has virtually no smell and keeps exceptionally well without going rancid, and, more important, without the need for artificial preservative. Any pulp left after the seeds have been pressed can be ground into a very nourishing flour possessing similar keeping qualities.

Sunflower meal and whole seeds were well known in Russia as a perfect way to bring domestic fowl into prime laying condition, and keeping them at peak lay for a whole season. Little did Russian peasants realize that, had they eaten the seeds direct or turned the meal into bread or biscuits, they would have had all the benefits of the seed protein without waiting for their chickens to lay eggs.

Cultivation of sunflowers has been carried on for many thousands of years, and there is some evidence that they were grown in large quantities by Amer ican Indians long before the pres ent tribal structure developed.

The stem, which can easily reach a height of 3m, is a masterpiece of natural structural engineering. The pith is surrounded by a strong tube of interlocked tissues, used in the past to make paper, and in China these were adopted to bulk out silk fibres for material stuffs.

When the plate-sized seed head is ripe it bends over to face the ground, and in the natural course of things, as the seeds dry they fall. To harvest your own sunflowers, cut the ripe seed heads from the stems and dry them in a current of air. They should not be hung in a shed or outhouse unless protected from damp, for although the seeds may be resistant to this the seed heads are not; they will quickly decay and impart a musty flavour to the seeds.

Certain therapeutic properties are contained in the oil. It is good for chest ailments and urinary disorders, though its action is extremely weak. However, the fact that the seeds are high in polyunsaturates makes them a good snack for anyone on a diet or with a high cholesterol level in their blood.

To roast or sauté a few seeds, put about 60g of kernels in a tablespoon of sunflower oil and cook until golden brown. Drain, and if your diet permits, roll them in salt and store in an airtight container until needed. The flavour is nutty and delicious and it's likely they won't remain in store for very long.

Sweet cecily
(Myrrhis odorata)
Family: UMBELLIFERAE

Few plants are so deserving of their common name as sweet cecily. Its name comes not as legend would have us believe from a beautiful woman, but from a corruption of the old English apothecary's Latin *sesli*, which is itself a corruption of the Greek word for a plant used in medicine.

The botanical name gives an indication of its properties, for it is indeed blessed with the pleasant odour of aniseed oil, and for sheer attractiveness there are few plants to rival its umbrella of white frothy flowers growing at the top of a stem decorated with feathery leaves of the brightest green. It grows in bushy clumps in early spring and keeps on growing until autumn.

Sweet cecily has been used medicinally for thousands of years, and the Greek physician Dioscorides recommended the whole plant as beneficial, from the flowers, which can be candied, to the roots, which can be cooked and eaten as a vegetable rather like potato.

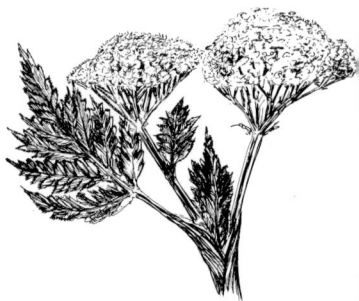

It has a considerable geographic distribution. North American Indians used it to soothe and charm horses; apparently they love the aniseed smell and taste. In France, leaves and smaller stems are dried and added to hops and other herbs as a pillow stuffing, and in the Middle Ages sweet cecily was used as a strewing herb for banqueting halls and for chambers frequented by the ladies of the castle.

Medicinally, it has many functions and few vices — so few, in fact, that from the Greeks onwards it was considered a plant that could not be overused.

Gerard was the first to adopt the name sweet cecily in print, and he recommended it either fresh or dried for constipation and as a general tonic.

When roasted, the strongly-flavoured seeds make an excellent appetizer with a little salt. The feathery leaves are at their best in spring and add extra flavour to ham sandwiches, while the crushed stems added to lemon juice drinks lessen the tartness.

One school of thought considers

the sugary sweetness of the stems beneficial to diabetics, for the actual sugar content is very low, and sweet cecily stems can be candied in much the same way as angelica.

It is an extremely useful and prolific herb for a herb garden. The flower heads should be picked as they appear or the plant will run to seed, causing the stems to become woody and the leaves tasteless.

Sweet woodruff
(Galium odoratum)
Family: RUBIACEAE

The most powerful herbs are often those that are the most insignificant to look at, and this is the case with sweet woodruff.

It's a woodland plant, as its name suggests, rather small and altogether unremarkable from its rough leaves to its small flowers which resemble those of the cuckoo flower, although they are unrelated. The stem is square, and the leaves that grow from each face are arranged in whorls said to resemble a wheel. This configuration is thought to explain the suffix 'ruff', the Saxon name being *wude rofe*, meaning 'wood wheel'.

The flowers have a pleasant scent which quickly fades when they are picked, and the stem and leaves are almost scentless when fresh. However, its fame as a strewing herb in castles during the Middle Ages was well earned, for when it's dried it gives off a scent of coumarin, the volatile ester which also comes from new-mown hay and sweet clover. Care needs to be taken when drying this herb, as fermentation can lead to toxicity if the plant does not dry properly.

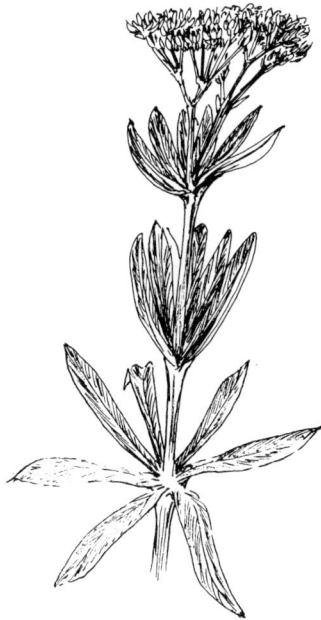

The depredations of clothes moths in a society whose garments were almost entirely composed of woollen fibres was drastic indeed, so the properties of woodruff were employed to protect and perfume clothes that had to be stored in closets and chests. There were few, if any, chemical moth repellants before the days of camphor crystals.

Woodruff and lavender were very popular because they do have a moth-repellent quality which operates by masking the smell of woollen cloth with heavy plant odours, fooling moths into thinking the clothes are really plant material. Woodruff has no insecticidal property as such.

Medicinally, it was highly praised for its ability to calm the nerves, in much the same way as modern tranquillizer drugs do today, except that modern drugs have considerable side-effects and are much stronger in their effect than infusions of woodruff. Gypsies adopted it as an ingredient in herbal teas for soothing the spirit. Although they were subjected to a hard life in Europe and Great Britain, the gypsies rarely suffered from mental disturbances.

Woodruff was well known to all ancient herbalists especially for its power to reduce the impact of liver infections, where it was either used as an internal medicine (a handful of dried herb in 1 litre of boiling water; 1 cupful taken 3 times a day), or applied externally as a poultice of fresh crushed leaves to treat the swelling of an enlarged liver.

The power of woodruff as a diuretic for reducing water retention is doubtful, as it is weak in action. More often it was used to lessen menstrual pains and to treat gynaecological infections, and at the same time to quieten the sufferer. There are references in some herbals to woodruff in treating postnatal depression, and for infections following the birth of a baby

in the less-than-hygienic conditions which prevailed prior to the First World War.

However, it is for its value as a tranquillizer that woodruff best deserves to be known. A pleasant way to prepare a tonic wine is to steep a handful of dried plant in half a litre of cheap sweet white wine for two weeks. Strain off the wine, which will now be flavoured with a pleasant taste of sweet woodruff. There may also be the beginnings of a secondary fermentation in the wine, making it slightly fizzy when stored for a few days in a tightly stoppered bottle (do not use screw-top bottles as pressure can burst them). This pleasant-tasting wine is taken in the morning, 1 small glassful per day, with gentle and effective results.

Tarragon
(Artemisia dracunculus)
Family: COMPOSITAE

USA: French tarragon

Tarragon is well known as a culinary herb, yet it also had a role in the herbal armoury of old. Sometimes known as French tarragon, it can be used to flavour vinegar. Steep a handful of dried leaves and twiggy stems in a litre of wine vinegar, preferably white. The taste is peppery with a hint of vermouth, not surprising when you consider that tarragon is a close relative of wormwood.

worst. At one time the twisted root of tarragon was chewed to ease the pain of toothache.

Two types of tarragon are generally available: Russian tarragon and the French variety. The Russian has less flavour but is far more vigorous; as its name implies, it is hardy, growing strong and tall, sometimes as much as 1m high.

The French variety is more refined and, being French, full of flavour and rather attractive, but not so vigorous; it needs plenty of sun to thrive. The flavour is a mixture of mild pepper and aniseed, one complementing the other, and the French consider egg dishes tasteless if tarragon is left out. It does have a distinctive taste, but it's doubtful if it would be absolutely essential for English palates.

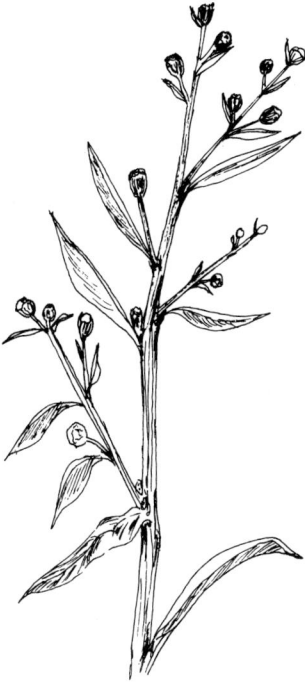

'Drago plant' is one of its old English names, because it was said to be a specific for snakebite and wounds caused by venomous creatures. It seems likely that this story was brought here by the crusaders in the Holy Land, for it appears that this plant species originally came from the Middle East and was recommended against the effects of scorpion stings.

Less dramatic is the use to which it is put in this country, to give relief from wasp stings, so make sure your tarragon plant is at its best when the wasps are at their

Thyme
(Thymus vulgaris)
Family: LABIATAE

USA: English thyme, French thyme

One of the oldest established culinary and medicinal herbs is the low-growing shrubby plant known as thyme. A particularly pretty story about this plant is that it appeared where Helen of Troy's tears fell to the stony ground, but the Greeks were using thyme long before the Trojan wars, and the Egyptians, too, made use of it.

It is a naturalized plant, probably brought over to Britain by the

Romans when they found that British native wild thyme (*Thymus serpyllum*) was too small and possessed too few of the active ingredients of *Thymus vulgaris*.

The thyme we grow in herb gardens today is very like the wild variety found growing in open areas in most Mediterranean countries.

Some hint as to its antiseptic abilities can be seen in the fact that it formed part of the compounds used by the Egyptians to embalm their dead, and thymol has been proved a powerful antibiotic when used in sufficiently high concentrations.

However, it was for the living that Romans imported it into England, specifically for culinary flavouring and the relief of flatulence and digestive upsets following the heavy meals that wealthy Romans loved to indulge in. Its capacity to soothe after an excess of eating made it famous, and its pleasant flavour ensured its popularity.

Thyme is best picked when in full flower to keep the active principles intact. It should be dried at a relatively low temperature out of the sun and in a very airy place. The tough foliage was evolved to prevent water loss, so the drying process can be lengthy. When dry, store in dark-glass jars with well-fitting lids in order to keep the dried plant from absorbing other undesirable odours.

Medicinally, an infusion of 1 tablespoon of dried thyme to a cup of very hot, but not quite boiling, water will yield a good calming drink, and if the taste is a little too strong, add a teaspoon of honey.

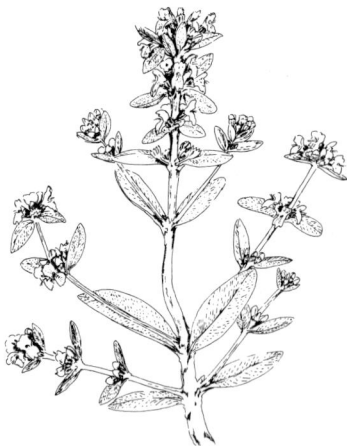

Coughs and colds are among the miseries that everyone falls prey to at some time or another, and the after-effects of a cold are almost as unpleasant as the primary infection. Sinus infections can be relieved by inhaling the vapours of two tablespoons of dried thyme in half a litre of water. This will also ease a tight chest and makes a good gargle for sore throats.

The advantage of using thyme as an inhalation is that it can be used twice. Once you have inhaled the steam, add a little marjoram, honey and a teaspoon of lemon juice, and it makes a beneficial drink to calm the digestive system and ease the discomfort that sometimes remains after a cold has abated.

Externally, an infusion of thyme

can be applied as a disinfecting wash for grazes or minor cuts, as the action of thymol on the skin is gentle. The addition of a sachet of thyme in the last jug of rinsing water when you wash your hair will leave your hair shining and with a pleasant clean smell too.

Valerian
(Valeriana officinalis)
Family: VALERIANACEAE

USA: garden heliotrope, valerian

In the countryside of fifty years ago valerian's pinkish flowers were a common sight in high summer, and their rather pungent smell attracted many bees, day-flying moths and small flies. Now it is less common, found in quantity only in the unspoiled parts of the west of England and South Wales.

In the past the Greeks were fond of using the dried root for treating nervous disorders and epilepsy, and it is as a sedative that it's best known. In fact, the commonest reference to valerian is as a herbal sedative.

The root is the part where medicinal power resides, and the smell of dried valerian root, which was used in the Middle Ages to protect clothes from moths, is generally accounted unpleasant. However, cats and rats are said to be irresistibly attracted to it, so its value as a protective agent for clothing stored in chests must be questionable, to say the least.

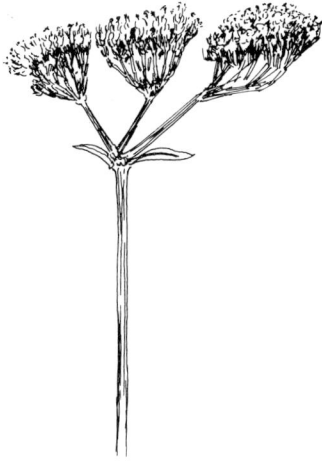

In the panic which followed the devastating outbreaks of bubonic plague in the thirteenth and fourteenth centuries all manner of herbal concoctions were made up in an attempt to provide an antidote, and as each outbreak occurred and the population became more and more frightened so charlatans went to work. Many 'remedies' were invented, and people were so desperate that they would try anything. Chaucer refers to valerian compounded with honesty (lunaria) but in fact this would have been quite useless for treating plague.

As a sedative valerian must be used with caution, for an overdose can cause symptoms of extreme anger, agitation and in rare cases delusions. There is a story that Adolf Hitler was a valerian addict, and he certainly displayed behavioural symptoms similar to those found with excessive use of this plant extract, though I can find no evidence to give substance to this tale.

Medicinally, the dried root, which as well as smelling foul also has an exceedingly bitter taste, is administered as a tincture for relieving nervous spasm, St Vitus Dance, and hysteria and convulsions in children. However, a word of warning here. Children's convulsions which sometimes occur with a high temperature should always be treated under the supervision of a doctor, as they can be a symptom of meningitis or some other disease that could lead to permanent disability or even death if not treated properly.

Nevertheless, if used properly the sedative effect of valerian can be of value. To make a night-time drink for temporary relief of sleeplessness, soak 10g of dried root in 1 cupful of cold boiled water for 8 hours, strain and take 1 tablespoonful in the afternoon and again before retiring for the night. Or take it in a tincture form, as available from qualified herbalists. The taste can be masked with honey and the addition of some fragrant herb such as chamomile, peppermint or balm.

Vervain
(Verbena officinalis)
Family: VERBENACEAE

USA: berbine, European vervain, herb of the cross, pigeon grass, simpler's joy

Of all the plants used by man to cure his ills, vervain appears to be one of the most widely employed and most highly respected, from the time of the Druids, who cleansed their altars prior to sacrifice with an infusion of vervain flowers, to the Romans who considered that it had the power to rekindle the fires of love, and indeed dedicated it to the goddess Venus and at New Year gave nosegays of the flowers to bring good luck and love in the year to come.

By early medieval times vervain was looked upon as a prime ingredient in love potions and philtres, and also as a charm against witchcraft and devils. It was said that children who wore a sprig of vervain would be good-humoured and quick to acquire knowledge, and rubbing the juice of vervain all over the body was supposed to be a sure way to obtain all the heart desired – obviously a reference to the plant's potential as a love potion.

Because vervain is so steeped in magic and ritual, it is hard to filter fact from fancy, but there is little doubt that the employment of vervain in treating difficult childbirth and as a styptic to staunch bleed-

effect on feverish headaches, being compared with quinine, and it is helpful too with indigestion, being a calming agent.

An infusion can be used externally for ulcers and is recommended for mouth ulcers and bad breath. There is also a treatment for rheumatism and lumbago which involves boiling a handful of vervain in a small amount of wine vinegar for a minute, then applying as a poultice as hot as bearable to the affected areas. This remedy is very popular in France.

Violet, sweet
(Viola odorata)
Family: VIOLACEAE

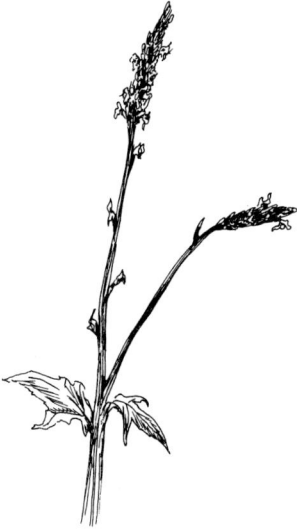

ing from deep wounds was widespread.

An infusion of 50g of dried plant to 1 litre of water, prepared by boiling for a few minutes and allowing to cool before straining, was generally prescribed all over northern Europe as a liver stimulant and for jaundice. One cupful 3 times a day was the prescribed dose. The same infusion was administered to relieve kidney infections and inflammation of the spleen.

One of vervain's constituents is a glucoside called verbenaline, credited with the power to reduce pain and fevers and relieve the symptoms of migraine headaches when associated with the onset of menstruation. An infusion of vervain does seem to have a beneficial

USA: English violet, March violet, sweet violet

'I think that the king is but a man, as I am; the violet smells to him as it doth to me.' So wrote Shakespeare in *Henry V*. This is just one of the many references Shakespeare made to violets. In *The Winter's Tale*, Perdita speaks of 'Violets dim, but sweeter than the lids of Juno's eyes', and this could well be a reference to the ancient Greek custom for women to paint their eyelids with purple sweet-scented ointment. The goddess Juno might have used such a cosmetic.

With its distinctive perfume and colour, sweet violet is well known throughout Europe, where it grows in the wild and as a cultivated plant. In the West Country a considerable cottage industry has been developed based on the perfume of Devon violets.

A plant of woodland and hedgebank, violets are one of the first flowers to bloom in spring, and are often confused with another member of the same family, dog violet, which is very similar but lacks the intense perfume, and has a lighter centre to its flower. The leaf is slightly different too, but these two plants, closely related to the ornamental garden flower heartsease or pansy, have medicinal as well as aesthetic values.

Since classical Greek times the leaves of sweet violets have been applied as an antiseptic for healing cuts and boils, containing as they do complex sugars called glucosides. The Greeks also used violets as a symbol of fertility, making the flowers into wine and confectionery, and they were followed in this by the Romans.

Violet petals can be made into a cough syrup and a tea to relieve bronchitis. The use of violets and another early flowering plant, coltsfoot, for relieving coughs, is well documented, but an infusion of coltsfoot, although effective, is nowhere near as pleasant as syrup of violets. In the past there was doubtless a distinction between violets for the lady of the house and coltsfoot tea below stairs.

In southern Europe the Romans brought the cultivation of the violet to a fine art, and large acreages were given over to its growth for wine and medicine. In the less salubrious climate of ancient Britain, young girls kept their skin in good condition with a lotion made from a mixture of goat's milk and violets. Bearing in mind the long winters living in damp smoke-filled huts, a lotion of violets must have made quite an improvement in both their appearance and their smell!

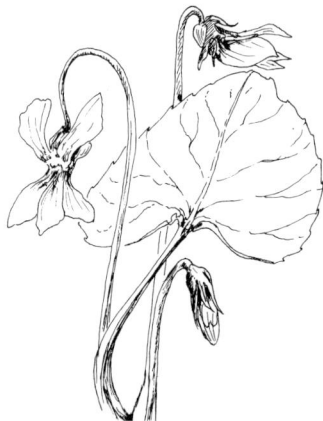

In the Middle Ages, however, monks were more interested in the violet's powers as a cure for insomnia, and also as a laxative. It was valued as a calming agent by the Victorians, too, who grew these attractive little flowers in their gardens as an ingredient for herb pillows.

Violet, dog
(Viola canina)
Family: VIOLACEAE

Dog violet was so called because it has no smell and was therefore considered to be of less value than sweet violet, but the plant has many of the medicinal virtues of its sweet cousin and they should be grown in a herb garden alongside one another.

In ancient times the leaves were eaten raw in salads and cooked in honey for their general tonic effect. Fresh leaves can be crushed and applied to bruises, wounds and abrasions, and the whole plant is dried and prepared as a tea for calming the nerves. There are many records in old herbals to the power of violets in epilepsy, to lift depression and generally to soothe the spirit.

Walnut

(Juglans regia)
Family: JUGLANDACEAE

Walnut is one of the most useful trees for furniture. It has the most attractive timber and formed the basis of the cabinet maker's art in England during the seventeenth century, preceding the Civil War.

It is at the northern limit of its climatic tolerance range in Great Britain, growing strongly only where rainfall is lower than average. Many large trees, now at the end of their lives, were planted at the instigation of monastic orders or in the grounds of convents for the nuts and medicinal products of the leaf and green outer casing of the shells.

The leaves are gathered just after they open, and when dried yield a blackish granule rather like some teas. This is recommended for dry skin and also skin eruptions.

Internally, a brew of 1 tablespoon of dried leaves to 1 litre of water is prescribed to reduce disorders of the digestive system, especially those associated with biliary imbalance. There are records of walnut infusions being employed to lower blood sugar

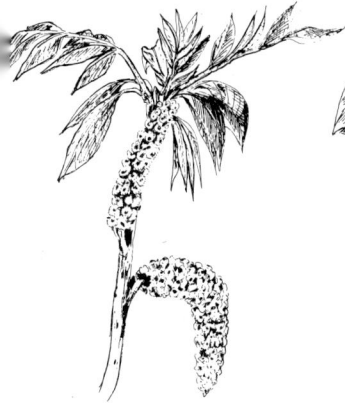

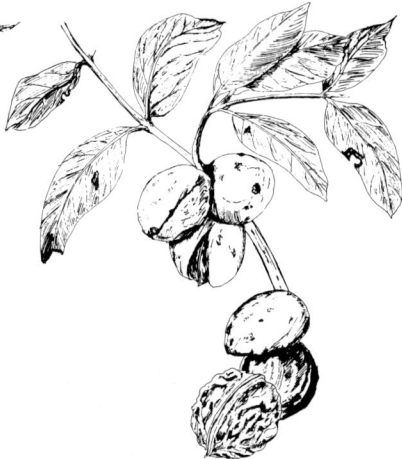

levels when treating diabetes, but far more effective drugs and regimes of diet are available to keep this disorder in balance. Walnut tea was drunk for gastro-enteritis and to dispel tapeworms. It is extremely astringent and not at all pleasant to take as an infusion.

Externally, the same brew can be used to bathe skin and reduce soreness or chafing. In the past several far-fetched claims for cures attributed to walnut leaves were made. One from France suggested they would cure cattle and men of the dreaded disease anthrax, but there is no evidence to prove this.

When preparing walnut shells and leaves in boiling water they give off a strong smell highly recommended for keeping flies and other biting insects at bay, though I've not tried it, for walnut juice can stain skin and clothes and it's not easy to get off.

Water agrimony
(Bidens tripartita)
Family : COMPOSITAE

When the science fiction novel, *The Day of the Triffids* came out it caused great interest and brought a new word for dangerous plants into the English language; 'triffid' became synonymous with menace. Yet the real 'triffid' is far from menacing, in fact it is a useful herb called water agrimony, trifid, or tripartite burr marigold, and there are a large number of closely re-

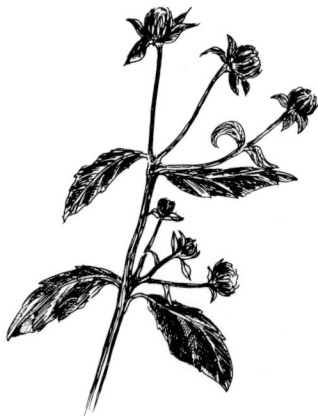

lated plants across all the temperate zones of Europe and North America.

It is found growing in ditches, on stream margins and at the side of quiet ponds and lakes. A member of the daisy family, it bears its yellowish button-like flowers at the top of tall smooth stems and when the flowers fade they are replaced by burr-like fruits which give the plant its name of burr marigold.

It has another name, hipatorium, indicating its use as a treatment for liver disorders and jaundice, and Culpeper mentions it in this context. He also refers to the fact that it was adopted as an infusion to relieve severe coughs and, as with most of Culpeper's favourites, it seems water agrimony was supposedly helpful in dealing with stones or gravel in the urinary tract. If Culpeper is to be believed, this was an exceedingly common ailment at the time of the Civil

War. Water agrimony was also recommended for treating worms.

Today water agrimony is confined to its use as a styptic for suppressing bleeding of the uterus and respiratory organs.

In North America a similar plant called swamp beggar's tick (*Bidens connata*) was also employed to suppress bleeding, and more especially to stem prolonged menstrual bleeding, the seeds being prescribed in powder form.

Leaves were applied to the head and chest of a patient as a hot fomentation to relieve congestion in cases of severe chest infection. Some of the uses to which swamp beggar's tick leaves were put appear rather cruel. Patients suffering with palpitations and croup were administered very strong doses at frequent intervals until they were forced to vomit, when they were considered to be cured. Records don't show how many people suffered lasting harm from such treatment.

Water lily

(Nymphaea alba)
Family: NYMPHAECEAE

Few water plants are more attractive than white or yellow water lilies. Over the years they have figured in many paintings, for artists have been inspired by the quiet tranquillity of this elegant denizen of lakes and gentle streams.

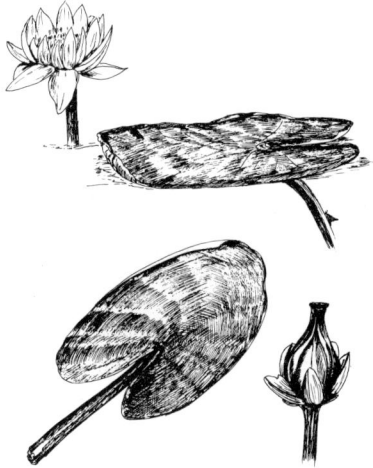

The Tale of Jeremy Fisher by Beatrix Potter would have been dull indeed without flat lily leaves to act as fishing rafts for the curious frog.

Water lilies will not grow where water runs frantically or where there is any sort of hustle and bustle. The water they favour must be pure and of a high alkaline level, and although their root systems are firmly in the ooze they keep their heads in the air.

Lilies have featured in stories and fables for generations, and the plant owes its family name to Greek water sprites. Legend has it they were great fans of the yellow lily (*Nuphar lutea*), which is a closely related species and is also known as the brandy bottle lily, for the flowers smell slightly of brandy and the seed vessel, when ripe, is similar in shape to the old-type brandy bottle.

Culpeper said of the water lily that 'it settles the brain of frantic persons', and it is taken nowadays as an anaphrodisiac or calming agent for reducing sexual desire.

There is a long association between water lilies and the organs of sexuality. When prepared as a lotion, the root was recommended as a vaginal douche, both internally and externally. The plant has considerable astringent powers, and probably some positive action against fungal spores in that it renders the area too acid for spores to germinate. It has been prescribed as an internal vaginal douche in the treatment of leucorrhoea, but this should be undertaken only under the guidance of a qualified medical practitioner. The danger of secondary infection, unless scrupulous standards of hygiene are followed, is extremely high. It is important to remember that our ancestors had considerable powers of recovery, and being exposed to many more ills than we have to face in our antiseptic society, their natural antibodies allowed them to pursue courses of treatment that would be unwise today.

However, for external use water lily root can be prepared for a lotion. Clean the root and grate into strips, then steep in boiling water for 10 minutes. The whole should then be raised to the boil and allowed to simmer gently for a further 10 minutes. Remove from the heat, keep covered and allow to cool before straining. Bottle for later use in tightly stoppered containers. It will keep for some time, but when opened should be used within a week. Any lotion remaining after this time should be discarded.

The lotion is recommended for treating skin irritations and sunburn, providing the skin is not broken, and for sores caused by abrasion. Fresh lotion is used as a gargle handy for sore mouths and gums.

To produce a poultice for boils and other such skin eruptions the root can be utilized in conjunction with slippery elm bark powder, and fresh young lily pads can be used as an emergency treatment for grazes. Bruise them and apply to the graze, binding with a cloth; change after three hours.

White bryony
(Bryonia dioica)
Family: CUCURBITACEAE

USA: bryony

This British member of a tropical gourd family has a host of common country names, quite a few of them referring to the poisonous qualities possessed by both berries and root. All in all, it is a plant best avoided.

Common in the south of England and the Midlands, white bryony is a scrambling climber of hedgerows and woodland margins, and its names of 'wood vine', 'wild hop', 'wood neps' and 'wild vine' allude to its powerful ability to climb and

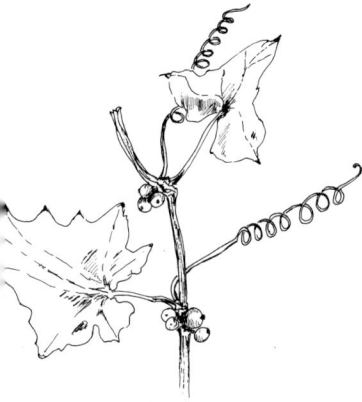

cover a hedge with grapevine-like leaves and tendrils.

White bryony flowers are green, insignificant things, but they drop soon after fertilization when the berries begin to develop. White at first, the berries redden at the end of August and at the same time the leaves begin to yellow at the edges.

The whole plant is sustained by a powerful root system which has led to other country names such as 'devil's turnip', and 'mandragora'. This latter came about because the root is large and sometimes grows to resemble a human shape. In the Middle Ages when mandrake root was employed in medicines and thought to have great powers, the substitution of bryony tubers for mandrake root was not uncommon, and the results of such a deception would almost certainly have been fatal. Bryony root contains toxic alkaloids and glucosides; the berries, too, contain similar poisons and are powerful enough to kill, just a handful of berries being sufficient to kill a child.

The incidence of poisoning by berries is luckily very rare, but parents are well advised to keep an eye on small children during blackberry-picking outings.

Medicinally, there are few uses for this plant except as a herbal tincture, when the dosage is so low as to be non-toxic.

In the Middle Ages bryony juice was employed only as a last resort on ulcers and skin eruptions that were not improving under normal treatment. Anyone having recourse to bryony would have suffered much discomfort, for juice made from the leaves and more particularly the root causes reddening of the skin after relatively short contact.

The Romans adopted the corrosive destructive nature of bryony as a means of removing warts and skin blemishes, and in seventeenth-century herbals it was recommended for removing freckles, but under no circumstances should bryony be used for this purpose. Contact with sensitive skins will almost certainly cause severe irritation and could well lead to scarring.

Wild arum
(Arum maculatum)
Family: ARACEAE

USA: dragonroot, Indian turnip
(A. triphyllum)

Every spring as the bluebells bloom so does another plant with a

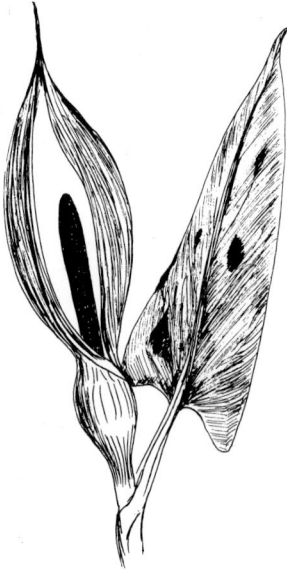

history almost as old as civilization in these islands. It is the cuckoo-pint, arum, or lords-and-ladies. These are just a few of the dozen or so names under which wild arum goes.

Despite the fact that the whole plant is poisonous, there are lists of diseases for which medieval herbalists believed it was the perfect treatment. As well as plague and a host of internal ailments, herbalists also recommended the root be exploited as a food, and there was a thriving trade in wild arum used in a dish called Portland sago or British arrowroot. When dried and ground to powder the flour is white and very fine, with a high concentration of starch; indeed, in country districts the plant is called 'starchwort' and 'wake robin', both terms for starching. It was employed in preparing ruffs and collars when they were in fashion in the sixteenth and seventeenth centuries.

Gerard noted that although it was a perfect starch, the hands of laundresses became cracked and damaged by toxins in the root, but despite this it continued in use until the Victorians refined other starches.

The flowers with their cowl-like leafy petals surrounding a central spike were known to children as red-hot pokers, and strangely enough the flowers do attract by the smell and heat generated by the spike. The pointed tip of the hood also helped to acquire for the arum another, much older, name of 'nedder's tongue', a corruption of the old English *nadderis*, the name for an adder.

It was said in Ancient Greece that the attentions of venomous snakes would be diverted from travellers who carried wild arum. Considering how few species of venomous snakes are found on the continent of Europe, even as far south as Greece, it is surprising just how many plants have been adopted as charms and proofs against snakebite. Many specifics are listed in medieval herbals in Britain, where you really have to work hard to get bitten by the only native poisonous snake, the adder.

These early herbals also stated that if you washed your hands in the juice of wild arum, snakes could be handled with impunity.

In fact there was far more danger from ingesting wild arum berries than from snakes; these berries are attractive to children and grow low down in woodlands, often under wild raspberry or blackberry bushes. They can be fatal if eaten in large quantities. Fortunately the berries are mainly purgative, and a child would most likely have little more than an extremely upset stomach for a few days, but it is wise to keep children under supervision when blackberrying, especially as that is the time when wild arum berries are most readily available to small hands.

In the Middle Ages the juice of this plant was distilled with milk and used to clear the skin. It was said to be a perfect way to reduce freckles. However, the likelihood of an allergic reaction is very real and it would be best to use the dried plant only under medical supervision.

Wild strawberry

(Fragaria vesca)
Family: ROSACEAE

There are still many places in our countryside where wild strawberries thrive, although excessive hedge trimming and destruction to create larger fields has removed much of the wild strawberry's habitat. They grow best in the West Country and in northern France, and propagate themselves by means of runners that can cover a considerable area. Cultivated strawberries were developed from this plant, but in the process lost some of the superb flavour of the wild berry.

Strawberries have considerable medicinal powers, and their usefulness in treating gout is well documented. The botanist Linné referred to strawberries as a blessing from the gods because he considered himself cured of gout by the expedient of eating large quantities of strawberries – a very enjoyable way to cure an unpleasant condition. Some sources state the exact opposite, however, so perhaps it might be better not to try this.

This plant contains many important constituents in its fruit, roots and leaves. One of them is salicylic acid, which some herbalists believe can have a beneficial effect on kidney function. It is valuable for lowering the body's uric acid levels, which in turn has a good effect on arthritis and rheumatism.

The fruit contains large quantities of iron in an easily assimilated form, and research is being carried out into reports that strawberry lowers blood pressure. It is useful for relieving gastroenteritis, helping to soothe and calm spasms of the gut. The fruit seeds are important too for healthy tone in the digestive system. They

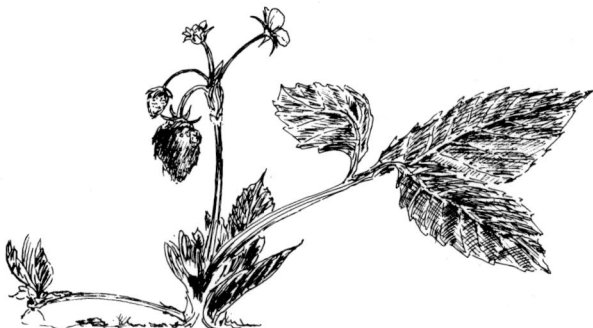

provide roughage and stimulate the bowel movement. However, the root is considered to be of greatest benefit for anyone suffering persistent gastritis or cystitis. It is dried and crushed and 25–30g of crushed root are boiled in 1 litre of water to which a cupful of chopped strawberry leaves has been added. The whole is boiled for 15 minutes, then strained and a little honey added to reduce the sharp taste. It makes an excellent health drink which is also good for a host of other ailments, including bronchitis.

A gargle for sore throats can be prepared from the leaves: 1 large cup of leaves to half a litre of water. Boil for 10 minutes, then strain.

Strawberry pulp has many uses externally and is often quite effective for the skin. However, some sensitive skins will react to it, so it's best to do a small test to check for reaction before attempting to apply it to your face.

One strawberry pulp remedy that I've come across is for treating chilblains, but I'm at a loss as to how this recommendation came about. Chilblains are normally a winter ailment and the availability of strawberries decreases dramatically with the onset of cold weather!

Willow

(Salix alba, Salix species, Salix fragilis)
(Pictured is 'pussy willow', Salix caprea)
Family: SALICACEAE

Long before aspirin tablets brought relief from headaches, willow and meadowsweet were used as a source of salicylic acid, the active ingredient in aspirin.

Quite a bit of research has been done in Europe into the active properties of willow, which contains salicylic aldehyde in the bark of the twigs.

All over the northern hemisphere willow bark used to be employed for treating the symptoms of head colds and influenza, but tannin, also present in the bark, gives any brew of willow bark a very astringent taste. Nevertheless, its ability to lower temperature and ease headaches and aching joints made this acceptable.

Now there are far more palatable ways of obtaining the active constituents in willow in tablet form, but as an emergency treatment whilst camping or walking, stripped willow twigs can give some relief. If steeped in boiling water for ten minutes they will yield enough active ingredients to salve a cut and reduce pain and swelling caused by wasp stings.

Bark should be gathered from twigs in spring and the most active bark is found on twigs that have been growing for between two and five years. After the bark has been stripped from the stems, a relatively easy process, it can be dried in the shade or in an airing cupboard and stored in dark-glass jars with tightly stoppered lids to keep it in prime condition.

Willow bark contains considerable quantities of tannin, and in the past five-to-ten-year-old branches were collected and used for tanning fine leather.

The lance-shaped leaves can be collected and dried, but they are low in salicylic aldehydes.

In recent years there has been increasing interest in aspirin for treating heart ailments and for relieving pain from inflamed rheumatic joints. It has the disadvantage that in refined form serious side-effects on the stomach lining may result. The far weaker

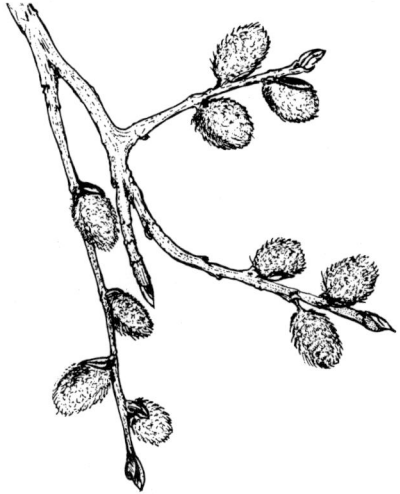

and naturally buffered qualities of willow may hold a key.

Powdered willow bark is excellent for relieving feverish cold and flu symptoms and if you want to try it take 2–3 tablespoons of powdered bark in 1 litre of hot water. It tastes astringent but is improved by adding marjoram. A cupful of this mixture is the usual dose 3 times a day.

Woody nightshade
(Solanum dulcamara)
Family: SOLANACEAE

USA: bittersweet

Woody nightshade is generally feared beyond its power, for although it is poisonous it is not as toxic as its near relative, belladonna or deadly nightshade.

Perhaps at blackberry-picking time when children are gathering the luscious fruit of the bramble there is a need to take care, as woody nightshade berries are temptingly red and grow in clusters often tucked in among the brambles. Taste is no deterrent, either, for the initial tartness of this member of the potato family changes to sweetness, hence the name 'bittersweet'.

The bitter flavour comes from an alkaloid glucoside called solanine found in the berries, and this is the same poison that gives belladonna its fearful power.

It is always most important to make sure children know which berries to pick and which to leave well alone. They could make a mistake and eat belladonna, in its red stage, with fatal results.

The family solanaceae is widespread, and many of its members are of value to man; the best-known is the potato. However, the berry of the potato, the potato apple, is poisonous, as are potatoes which have turned green through exposure to daylight. The poisonous substance liberated is oxalic acid, a powerful corrosive toxin that will react with rust on metal to form a skin of metallic salts. These salts were used by ancient gunsmiths to colour gun barrels and the blades of expensive swords.

Woody nightshade is a common plant of disturbed ground, and when established in an allotment it's extremely difficult to eradicate without recourse to strong and undesirable chemicals. Its many country names include 'felon herb' and 'felon wort', allusions to its toxic properties. Another, 'woodbine', describes the way the tendrils wind around like honeysuckle bines. Other names such as 'dulcamara' and 'mortal' ascribe properties more akin to witchcraft than herbal folklore, and 'violet bloom' comes from the beautiful violet-coloured flowers which appear in clusters throughout the fruiting season. The flower is similar in shape to that of the tomato, also a member of the same family.

The leaves of bittersweet boiled in wine may be used externally to reduce swelling caused by sprains, and both shoots and leaves can be employed to soothe external haemorrhoids. However, to my mind this condition is too serious to treat with home-made remedies and any

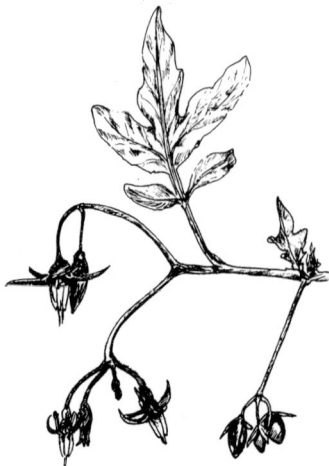

medicaments should only be used after consulting a qualified medical practitioner.

All in all, it is really best for amateurs to avoid this plant; there are too many potential hazards from its misuse.

Yarrow
(Achillea millefolium)
Family: COMPOSITAE

USA: milfoil, nosebleed, yarrow

The Greek warrior Achilles was said to have used yarrow to heal his companion's wounds, and the feathery leaves of this common wayside herb have been employed in this way for centuries all over Europe. Its Latin name denotes the 'thousand cuts' in the leaf, and it's rich in country names, 'millfoil', 'thousand leaf', and 'nosebleed' being just a few.

As well as being a medicinal herb, it's a welcome addition to meadowland flora, where it's a popular fodder plant. Horses will eat it readily and its aromatic foliage gives a distinctive odour to hay. The flowers are similar to the heart of a small cauliflower, being closely packed, and are pink or white in colour with each tiny flowerlet having a yellow centre.

The leaves and flowers can be used either fresh or dried, but they ought not to be dried in direct sunlight, for as with most aromatic herbs the oils – the active constituent of the plant – will be destroyed or evaporate.

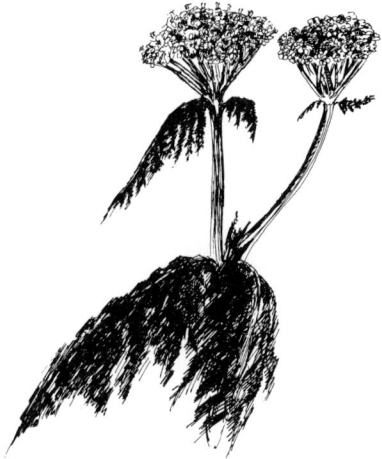

As well as weapons of war, our forefathers were surrounded by edged tools of lethal design. It is fairly unusual nowadays to see severed fingers and other mutilations caused by tools and machinery, but it was quite a different case just a few generations ago. This in part accounts for the wide range of herbs used to staunch blood flowing from open wounds, and yarrow, being common, was widely available.

A drink prepared from 50g of yarrow to 1 litre of cold water, brought to the boil and then stood for 10 minutes to infuse was recommended for stomach cramps, and this remedy was also prescribed to reduce bleeding and subsequent anaemia in haemorrhoid sufferers and to alleviate menstrual haemorrhage. Yarrow should never be used during pregnancy.

Growing and Cultivation

One point to remember when sowing wild plants for herbal medicine is that some of them will be much more successful if they have little or no competition from grasses and other ground-cover plants, as anyone who has grown mint in a fertile border will testify.

Mint soon takes over the entire area unless controlled in a confined space such as a bucket with the bottom removed. A deep ring-culture sleeve sunk into the soil will prevent the root systems of vigorous plants going where they're not wanted.

Many wild plants and herbs are intolerant of artificial fertilizers and very susceptible to weedkillers; even the residue in a well-washed sprayer can do irreparable harm, and after all the very reason for growing medicinal herbs in your garden is to ensure a clean and uncontaminated supply.

Most culinary herb seeds are available from top-quality specialist garden centres and smaller nurserymen, who tend to specialize in the unusual. Always plant as instructed.

Many wild plants are also available as seeds from garden centres, and those plants protected by law are often supplied as seeds from garden-grown stock. Do not be tempted to go into the countryside and uproot species for your garden. There is no excuse for putting our natural flora under any extra pressure.

One of the joys of growing medicinal plants is that when you tell your friends you often find they are of a like mind. Soon you will have seeds and cuttings, roots and tubers offered to you from the most unlikely gardeners. Then it will not be a case of what is available, but one of where you can find the space to plant them all.

It is most enjoyable and rewarding to grow your own medicinal herbs, propagating them from seed or root cuttings. One golden rule to follow to ensure effective germination, is always to try to duplicate in a seedbed conditions as close as possible to the plant's natural habitat.

Many seeds need a period of low temperature and dormancy to ensure they germinate when spring arrives, especially members of the primula family like cowslips and primroses; and most naturally occurring plants in the United Kingdom, northern Europe, mountainous areas of southern Europe and much of temperate North America require a cold, damp resting time.

If you experience difficulty in getting native species to germinate, put the seeds in a refrigerator for four weeks, packed in a little damp sterilized soil or damp sand, then sow them in the usual way in seed trays in a cold greenhouse or in the garden in prepared beds.

Of course, some wild plants are the very opposite of reticent, and to ensure your herb garden is not overrun with one species always start off seeds in seed boxes, either indoors or outdoors depending on time of year and species, then thin out and give any left over to other herb gardeners of your acquaintance.

Proprietary seed composts are often the most satisfactory way of ensuring your seeds start life in the safest, most sterile conditions, but remember that native plants suffer fewer pests and diseases than introduced species.

Try never to use sprays, chemicals or fertilizers. They leave harmful residues or noxious chemicals on the foliage and in tissues and roots.

Some plants have strict soil requirements, but the joy of a herb garden is that you can put them where you need them simply by preparing the ground for their particular needs. For instance, both lime-loving and acid-tolerant species can be planted in the same bed by providing soil of the correct acid or alkaline balance in large 'culture rings', available from nurserymen for growing melons or tomatoes. Various species of mints can be contained in the same way. This will allow certain less vigorous types of mints, especially peppermint, which can lose out to spearmint, to grow happily in one small area without root competition for vital nutrients.

These plastic rings can be buried to ground level and the spaces between filled with ground-covering aromatic herbs such as chamomile lawn, which gives off a pleasant smell when crushed. I wouldn't advise pennyroyal for infilling, because being a mint species it will invade areas reserved for other herbs. Chamomile lawn tends to be less invasive and slower-growing and therefore easier to keep in check.

Choice of plants for your herb garden is an individual thing and there may be some you wish to cultivate which are not listed in this book. Space and personal inclination will dictate this, but one thing is absolutely certain: you will want to add to or change some plants over the years, so don't plan a garden that is too rigid in shape or form. One other advantage of ring cultures is that they allow you to add or subtract any species more easily.

Formal or informal also depends on your taste, and on the amount of land at your disposal, but remember that insects, butterflies, moths and birds will make use of your garden, too, and this is a wonderful opportunity to plant species for the benefit of nature. Nettles are less than welcome in most gardens, but you could grow a patch just for butterflies to lay their eggs on, and then you will have nettles for nettle beer and as a vegetable in spring.

In planning the layout, make sure you put the tall species such as fennel and sweet cecily where they won't shade out less vigorous species or grow across the garden path. Fennel can reach nearly $2\frac{1}{2}$m and cover a considerable area.

Always grow those plants that interest you. Do not be bound by any hard-and-fast rules. Many people have a border to spare, but others have to be content with pots and window boxes. Even these can prove excellent for all but the tallest varieties.

Plan your herb garden around culinary herbs initially, for all culinary herbs have medicinal properties. Mints of as many species as space allows are essential, and pay particular attention to peppermint, spearmint and orange or eau-de-cologne mints, for these have a variety of uses. Garlic and chives are also essential, as are thyme, sage and marjoram.

Fennel is limited in use and also occupies a great deal of space, but it is extremely attractive for a larger garden. Sweet cecily is a must, for the stems are edible as well as the foliage, and its virtues for the digestion make it popular. Borage is an attractive plant for the medical section of your herb garden, but comfrey tends to be better for a larger bed, as it is a vigorous plant with limited use. Its properties for healing ulcers and knitting bones are not often required, and it can shade a large area of a small flowerbed.

If you have a large area it is well worth including coltsfoot, a plant that can be difficult to propagate in gardens, but is handy. Do also try to grow meadowsweet; it will take two years to flower from seed. Along with a small pot-grown weeping willow this will give you the raw material for a herbal headache remedy, and both plants are popular with insect visitors. Don't plant willows close to your house unless they are in containers, for they are waterside inhabitants and will block drains and damage foundations as their roots search for water.

There are any number of plans for herb and physic gardens, from pathside to wheel-shaped, oblong to square, ground-level and raised by brick or stone containing walls. However, I think the only way to plan a really effective garden for both medicinal and culinary plants is to have one that fits its surroundings and your personal requirements. Do leave yourself a measure of flexibility, though, as you'll be bound to want to expand as your interest in the subject of herbal medicine increases.

Note
If you are interested in attracting butterflies to your garden as well as growing herbs and medicinal plants, listed here are a few species well loved by butterflies:

Primrose	Lavender
Alyssum	Catmint
Thrift	Hyssop
Honesty	Verbena
Valerian	Golden rod
Bugle	Sweet rocket
Sweet william	

GATHERING

There are many old wives' tales about the most propitious time to pick herbs and medicinal plants. The midsummer solstice was always reckoned a good time and tied in with old religious festivals that somehow became absorbed into the folklore of the Christian church, when it supplanted Druidic cults of tree- and nature-worship.

It just happens that midsummer is an excellent time to collect plants for drying, for despite the vagaries of our climate we usually enjoy a spell of calm hot weather then and plants most used for herbal preparations are at their best at this time. From the beginning until the middle of July they are in peak condition.

Collecting plants can have its hazardous moments: hemlock (*Conium maculatum*) is a case in point. Throughout the ages this relative of parsley and hogweed has commonly appeared at the edge of streams and many other wet and poorly drained places. Children are often the victims of hemlock poisoning, cutting the hollow mottled stems for pea shooters. Very small amounts of the alkaloid poison will cause death, and all parts of the plant are dangerous, particularly because they resemble other innocuous members of the same family.

The advice of a reliable botanist is an insurance policy for your safety, and it's a good idea to make contact with your local Naturalists' Trust, whose address will be in the telephone directory. They will welcome your support and you will benefit from their guidance.

Apart from saying that it is unwise to collect plants from the side of busy roads because of contamination, I would mention that many small undisturbed lanes are full of plants. They should be collected in the fullness of the day after the dew has dried and when any surface water will have evaporated. This last fact is very important, for the enemy of dried plant materials is water and mould growth, as they break down the cellulose structure.

I like to imagine in my mind's eye the Druids of old scouring the countryside on Midsummer's Day for those plants that would see them through the year's ills and help with a few spells as well, for they were as much concerned with myth and magic as with fact and medicine. Then as now, they needed to pick plants in their prime, choosing the flower at the point of opening or when the shoot was at its maximum growth point, and picking unmarked, unblighted leaves, rejecting those that aphids had made sticky and diseased.

As a final note, if any member of your family suffers from allergic reactions or hay fever, check they are not made unwell by your plants. The pollen of some very ordinary plants such as dandelion is a common allergen, and if hay fever sufferers are exposed to it for long periods the reaction to the allergen becomes progressively more severe.

Preparation of Plants

It is all very well having collected and dried your herbs and plants, but with such a cornucopia of potential medicine, most important of all is how to prepare them.

Tinctures, essential oils, oils, dried herbs, lotions and teas are all traditional ways of preserving and using herbs and flowers and as such have stood the test of time. From the eighteenth century onwards, preservation by low temperatures was also possible.

Drying

The preparation and storage of herbs is of paramount importance. If this simple aspect is carried out incorrectly then all your efforts will have been in vain, and on opening your jars of herbs, gathered with such enthusiasm during summer, you will find a rather musty-smelling collection of mouldy hay with no medicinal or even aesthetic appeal.

Methods of drying herbs vary wherever the art of herbalism is carried on in the world, but there are a few important rules to follow if you are not to waste time and plants.

Drying on netted racks is one of the best ways of ensuring plant material remains in perfect condition. You can make up trays from nylon net or muslin stretched over a wooden frame. This is a good use for all those old or damaged picture frames you can pick up at jumble sales for a few pence, and nylon net is cheap enough in most dress material shops.

These frames allow air to circulate freely, so that drying can take place quickly before moulds form. It is essential, too, that any drying area is free of strong aromas. I'm thinking particularly of the all-pervading smell of petrol that will contaminate the air in a garage and certainly be picked up by some of the more delicately flavoured plants; flowers especially will absorb strong smells.

Some plants used for culinary and medicinal purposes are woody and hard to dry, while others, mostly those originating from sub-tropical regions, are adapted to dry conditions and will take forever to dry if not assisted by some means of artificial heat. For instance, rosemary and thyme are both shrubby with leaves that will resist dessication. Lavender, too, can lose some of its fragrance if allowed to air-dry in daylight.

Flash-dry flower petals in hot sun for a few hours, then finish off in the shade to preserve colour. Raspberry leaves and many others such as walnut or lime should be initially dried in the sun and then finished to full dryness in a shed or an airing cupboard. For these particular plants it's best to use a drying frame in an airing cupboard. Space in an airing cupboard is usually at a premium in today's compact houses, however, and it would be unwise to dry all aromatic herbs in this way as some can transfer their smell to material fibres, not always with pleasant results.

The temperature of any cupboard you do use should not rise above 140° Fahrenheit (60° centigrade), or many of the properties of more delicate herbs such as eau-de-cologne or orange mint will be destroyed. However, others such as sage could almost be dried in an oven.

One sure tip to remember if you don't know whether it is safe to dry a particular herb in the sun is to find out if the plant grows best in full sun or in the shade. If in the shade, such as woodland-edge plants like elderflower, then dry it out of full sunlight.

The enemy of herbs is damp and mould. Flower preparations are totally destroyed in a few weeks if not completely dry. Some chemists' shops and wine-makers have silica gel dessicant sachets to ensure the keeping qualities of your precious plant substances by absorbing any moisture present in the jar where herbs are stored.

Perhaps the oldest method of drying herbs and medicinal plants is to hang them up in an airy place, and most plants dry very well if tied into bunches and hung in the shade. One or two tips will ensure the end result is as perfect as you can make it.

With due regard to the original quality of the plant material and how it is gathered, before any herb is hung for drying it should be absolutely surface-dry, free of raindrops and dew.

To make up bunches for drying, spread plants out on a sheet of clean greaseproof paper and remove any creepy-crawlies. Shake them back out into the garden; they will soon find new homes. Gather up bunches of six to ten stems depending on the size of plant; for example ten stems of mint makes a satisfactory bunch, whereas only six stems of valerian or mugwort are needed.

Bind the stems tightly at their woody ends with plastic-coated garden wire. They will shrink as they dry and the advantage of garden wire is that you can tighten the bunch by making another turn around the stems.

Hang these bunches on a 'clothes line' of garden wire in an airy shed or some other dry airy place with no strong smells such as petrol or solvents. If the weather is good your bunches will be dry enough for storage in about two weeks. Check for dryness by crumbling a leaf or two in your hand and if the plants are dried exactly right they will retain much of their original colour and most of their properties.

The golden rule is: take time and avoid strong sunlight. Results will be near-perfect herbs for storage and use.

Preparing teas

You will read about tisanes, teas, macerations, brews, and as many titles for concoctions as there are hairs on a gooseberry, but in essence there are very few basic methods that have stood the test of time since the Chinese and Egyptians prepared their medicines and unguents thousands of years ago.

The simplest and one of the most useful is a tea, prepared either by adding plants to boiling water and soaking them, or by bringing water to the boil with plants already in it.

Chamomile, marjoram, mint and balm make excellent teas and should be prepared in the normal way, with water added to the plant at the moment of boiling in order that water and heat can combine to extract the maximum benefit.

Any bowl, dish or jug in which the brew is prepared should be pre-heated, as this will allow the heat to be retained by the water and not transferred to the cold container. Containers should also be covered to retain volatile vapours that would otherwise escape into the air.

Containers should be of heat-proof glass or glazed earthenware, or if you have no other heat-proof material of the right size or shape, a stainless-steel saucepan can be used. Don't use iron or aluminium utensils for brews, as this often produces an unpleasant metallic taste and certain high-tannin-content plants can affect the surface of the saucepan. It is also most unwise to use plastic containers, for the faint taste of solvent that always remains even in the best-quality plastics can be amplified by aromatic oils in the herb.

The vapours of some plants, especially marjoram, mint and thyme, can be of value to people who suffer from catarrh. A mixture of these plants pounded in a bowl to release the essential oils of thymol and menthol and then allowed to stand in boiling water will produce a vapour that can be inhaled and often proves very soothing to mucous membranes of the nose and throat.

A word of caution here. It is easy to scald the delicate skin just inside the nose if you inhale too deeply or too close to the liquid. Put the hot brew in a tall heated jug and inhale the vapours carefully from under a towel.

Freezing

During the Regency period, a time of flowering for culture and scientific medicine, physicians realized that many ills of the time were due not to ill humours or miasmas but to more tangible things like moulds and bacteria, and though they were unsure of the origin of many diseases they understood that food remained wholesome for longer if it was cooled below the normal freezing point of water.

The ability to produce such temperatures mechanically was beyond their technology, but they capitalized on the naturally occurring cold of mid-winter and stored ice at low temperatures in multi-cavity insulated ice houses buried beneath the soil. Many of these ice houses still exist in the grounds of great houses, although now they are redundant structures where wintering bats hibernate. As low temperature stores, however, they were very effective.

The ice, gathered in deepest winter from frozen ponds and

lakes, stayed solid until summer, but still it was impossible to deep-freeze plants as modern technology has allowed us to do. Nowadays even the most ordinary low-temperature refrigerator or domestic freezer is capable of preserving herbs and plants for several months almost in the same condition as when they were picked.

However, there is a misconception that the domestic deep-freeze will generally maintain vegetable matter in good condition for far longer than is actually the case. The practice of blanching also often destroys the medicinal value of delicate foliage. A better method of preserving plants in a freezer for a considerably longer period, possibly even until the next growing season, is as follows:

Wash and dry herbs to eliminate external contamination. Prepare 1 litre of freshly boiled water, allow to cool and cover with a clean cloth. Put it in the freezer so that ice crystals just begin to form. When this happens take it out of the freezer and dip the clean dry herbs into it, then put them back into the freezer, where they will become glazed with ice and sealed against dessication.

The glazed herbs should be packed in tightly sealed freezer bags in small quantities until required.

Lastly, as with all preservation of medicinal plants, there is little use in carefully tending them if when you come to use them you can't identify them. All plants should be carefully and clearly labelled.

However, although misidentified plants can be an annoyance, they should never be dangerous. It is foolish in the extreme to fill your freezer with plants you know to be toxic or of which you are unsure. The object of herbal medicine is gentle healing, so gather only those plants you know to be safe.

Preparation in alcohol

For many years brews and teas were the only way the majority of herbs could be administered, and in consequence a large number of potent ingredients remained unused because they were insoluble in water.

Many plants have constituents as oils and gums that will combine with alcohol or olive oil. Quite a few of the French and Italian herbalists still use Roman remedies, derived from the Greeks who in turn gathered their information from the Arabs and

Egyptians, who had contact with the Chinese via the silk routes of the East. Eastern pharmacopoeias preserved essential oils and herbs in strong wines.

One of the problems of brewing herbs to be taken internally is that invariably you tend to make far more than you can use, and while some herbs will keep for a week, the average recommendation is no longer than three days, even in a refrigerator.

The herbalist's curse is fermentation, a problem we still find today, although this can be turned to advantage if you want to produce wines from plants like elder or some other fruit with a high sugar content.

Left to itself in a reasonably warm atmosphere, one of two things will happen to a preparation of plants that has been brewed in water. Firstly, it will begin to ferment and fine bubbles will appear to cloud the glass. Then, if fermentation is allowed to continue and there is very little sugar present to inhibit organisms, a mould will develop, very similar in form to penicillin.

Alcohol, a by-product of yeast fermentation, is one of the oldest and most powerful antiseptics known to man and has been around for many thousands of years.

To my knowledge there are no living organisms, plant or animal, that are not killed by alcohol. Even yeast itself, despite a natural tolerance to the compound, is eventually destroyed by it. Were this not so, then wine and other fermented drinks could be made as strong as whisky merely by the addition of larger quantities of sugar to the must – the term used to describe fermenting liquid.

Because this is not so, alcohol has to be concentrated and purified by distillation achieved by bringing the wine or mash containing the dilute alcohol to a temperature where it is boiled off, leaving the rest of the liquid in the vessel. Alcohol is then condensed from a vapour into liquid by cooling, and the resulting concentrated alcohol bottled. Depending on the raw material, skill and method applied, it ends up either as commercial alcohol or the finest brandy or malt whisky.

Alcohol has two properties which interest herbalists. Firstly, it is a powerful preservative, and a product mixed with a suitable strength of alcohol in a permanently sealed non-porous vessel will keep almost indefinitely. Secondly, it is a solvent for many of the gums, waxes and essential oils in which the healing properties of many herbs are vested. Essences of herbs in alcohol are known as tinctures, and tinctures of herbs are widely used in herbal medicine and homoeopathy, where dosages are minute and it's necessary to keep the mother tincture for some considerable time.

Alcohol is a proscribed product in its pure form and only a chemist is permitted to prescribe it in preparations. Therefore if you wish to prepare your own tincture you will have to use a proprietory spirit that does not have a flavour of its own. Vodka or aquavit are suitable, though the concentration is less than commercial alcohol.

Crushed plant material should be put into a glass container, about three-quarters of its volume. Add alcohol to fill the container. Seal to prevent any evaporation of spirit, and stand it in bright sunlight for two weeks. If this spirit tincture is not strong enough, pour off the liquid, press the plant material to recover the remaining spirit and add to a fresh quantity of plant. Repeat the process for a further two weeks. One of the best herbs to begin with is eau-de-cologne mint.

After all this you should have a tincture that can be used for external purposes.

Tinctures are interesting to produce, but you usually end up with far too much and they are readily available from a qualified herbalist, homoeopath or herbal supplier.

Preserving in oils
One of the most popular ways of preserving active ingredients of herbs for future use is to extract the principles in oil. Many recipes call for olive oil because it was one of the few oils available in the past, but it has been proved by time and usage to be the best. Other refined oils such as corn oil will do, but the best substitute for olive oil, and one that has added benefits, being high in polyunsaturated fats, is sunflower seed oil.

Confusion can occur between the terms 'oils' and 'essential oils' when discussing plant extracts. Some plant oils are volatile and can be distilled with heat, but generally this process is too dangerous, too expensive or simply too time-consuming and difficult for amateurs to undertake. Anyway, these distilled oils are usually available at reasonable cost from reputable herbal suppliers.

The method of extracting active principles in oil is sometimes called maceration, a term I find less than expressive for the combination of olive oil, plant, and the action of heat and/or sunlight to extract medicinal virtues.

To prepare an oil from a plant, it is necessary to crush or pound fresh or dried plant, depending on variety and directions in the original recipe, into small pieces. Put into a clear-glass jar, one that has a tightly fitting lid – a kilner jar is ideal. The jar should be filled with plant material and then olive oil or sunflower seed oil carefully poured over it until all the spaces are filled with oil. It is astonishing just how much oil a seemingly full jar of plant material will hold. When the jar is almost full, put the lid on and shake. This will allow the oil to penetrate the plant fibres and dispel any bubbles of air. Top up with additional oil if needed and reseal.

Leave the jar on a window-sill in bright sunlight for at least a month, or longer if the weather is dull. As it settles add more plant and oil. After a month, press the contents and strain off the oil. Add to a second jar of plant material and stand for a further four weeks. This will concentrate active ingredients or scent and flavour, whichever property is desired.

This method also applies to sweetly scented herbs such as lavender and mints, although they require frequent addition of fresh plant material if they are to develop sufficient strength or flavour. Marjoram and rosemary also both yield excellent flavoured oils.

Plants used to treat skin abrasion and infections are frequently prescribed in oil, especially St John's wort.

Most oils have good keeping qualities, especially those prepared with olive oil.

Bees and Honey

No book on herbs would be complete without a reference to bees, for without them few herbs would be pollinated and set seed. Prior to the advent of cane and beet sugar bees provided the main source of sweetening, namely honey.

A swarm of bees in May is worth a load of hay;
A swarm of bees in June is worth a silver spoon;
A swarm of bees in July is not worth a fly.

This little rhyme is one of many old sayings about the countryside that will be familiar to any beekeepers among you. Beekeeping must be one of the oldest forms of man's exploitation of nature, and these days it is carried out so that colonies are able to survive the winter. The keeper takes the honey store for his own use, or for sale, but makes sure that the bees have enough food in the form of sugar syrup to see them through winter. This was not so in the old days when every cottager had his 'skip' or 'skep' of bees in the garden, a romantic edifice of plaited, twisted straw that gave our language the word 'beehive', now used for any item so shaped. In those days many colonies were killed, smoked over a fire inside their hives. Although this was wasteful, the cottager couldn't afford to provide for them until the following spring.

Smoke is still used in beekeeping to stupefy the insects so that combs can be gathered from the frames that hang inside box-shaped modern hives, like so many books in a rack.

A bee is a very economical flyer, doing about seven million miles to the gallon (of honey, that is) and in order for a bee to gather a pound of honey it would have to travel roughly the equivalent of three times around the world on its journey from flower to flower.

Honey has long been used as a sweetener, a preservative, a medicine and a drink. It has been employed to preserve a multitude of foods, and Ancient Egyptians placed it in containers in the tombs of their kings, where traces of the sugary compound have remained. Honey has the power to inhibit growth of moulds and bacteria, and because of this property it was often used as a dressing for wounds, where it acted as a barrier between open vulnerable flesh and the contaminating air until the body's own healing power could do its work.

Being a natural sugar, honey is a good preservative, and many herbals recommend it to enhance the taste of plants with a high tannin content such as raspberry. However, honey is high in calories and ought to be avoided if you're on a strict calorie-controlled diet.

Beeswax, too, forms the basis of many herbal remedies, where it has much the same property as honey, acting as an air-proof barrier, but still allowing the moisture in the skin to evaporate. Beeswax is a very complex substance, and some that was applied to furniture in the sixteenth century is still intact. It was for treating wood rather than treating wounds that beeswax was best known, but the main purpose of this almost indestructible wax was for candles for the Church and nobility – few peasants could afford beeswax candles. Commoners would have to be content with the smoky flame of a rush soaked in tallow, or if things had gone well in the strip lynchet that year, then perhaps a tallow candle would light the family's evening activities.

When the comb had been crushed and the last of the old stocks of honey squeezed out, the wax was washed and the washings, if not boiled to crystallize the remaining honey, were allowed to ferment with fruit and water to make mead, or megethlin, as it was more commonly known. Mead was drunk in Viking halls, and pretty foul stuff it must have been. They didn't wait for it to mature but drank it when still hazy after fermentation, before the honey taste had modified. Anyone who has made mead will know that it tastes like sweet pond water until it is at least six months old. It is said that mead is not really drinkable for seven years.

Until the taste of honey fades to be replaced with a sherry-like mellowness, mead is not at its best.

In recent years the virtues of royal jelly have been much advertised. Royal jelly is a refined mixture of honey pollen and bee hormones that worker bees provide as food to certain bee grubs. These grubs develop into queen bees and found new colonies, but if they don't have this special diet they metamorphose not as fertile queens, but as humble infertile worker females. Although there is little evidence to prove or disprove the efficacy of royal jelly, many who have eaten it claim wondrous results. However, there is always the possibility that greater care in their diet as a whole may account for any improvement.

General Information

There have been drastic changes in our countryside since the days when herbal remedies were the only means available to treat some ills. Rough land and common were the herbalist's medicine chest, but now most of these have been cultivated or treated with fertilizers that have altered their herbage. These changes have left roadside banks as the main repository of many plants, but contamination is likely, so it's far safer to purchase your herbs from a recognized herbalist.

The Herb Society was formerly known as The Society of Herbalists and they provide an information service. The address is 34 Boscobel Place, London SW1 9PE. Send s.a.e. with your enquiry; this speeds up the service no end.

The professional body of medical herbalists belong to The National Institute of Medical Herbalists: General Secretary, Mrs Janet Hicks, 41 Hatherley Road, Winchester, Hants. Send them a large s.a.e. for a regional list of practical medical herbalists.

Other addresses that may be of interest are:

The Institute for Complementary Medicine, 21 Portland Place, London W1N 3AF.

The School of Herbal Medicine Phytotherapy, 148 Forest Road, Tunbridge Wells, Kent TN2 5EY.

The British Homoeopathic Association, 27a Devonshire Street, London W1.

Interesting and informative leaflets on herbal medicine can be obtained free from Holland & Barrett health food shops; you can just pop in and pick one up.

Mail-order services for obtaining herbs seem to be a good idea. Addresses to write to are:

Herbs By Post, The Barn, Wellesbourne Road, Moreton Morrell, Warwick CV35 9DB.

Herb Trade Association, Reg Peprow, 46 Church Street, Buckden, Huntingdonshire.

Lighthorne Herbs, Lighthorne Rough, Moreton Morrell, Warwick.

Certain organizations work for the health and well-being of the natural world, especially naturally occurring plants, and before attempting any explorations into the flora of the United Kingdom it is an excellent idea to be aware of existing legislation.

The Nature Conservancy Council, PO Box 6, Godwin House, George Street, Huntingdon, PE18 6BU, was established by act of parliament in 1973 and is the body appointed by the government to promote an understanding of nature conservation. They publish pamphlets as guidelines for many official and unofficial bodies; one entitled *Wildlife, the Law and You* is an invaluable guide to the Wildlife and Countryside Acts regarding conservation legislation.

They support and maintain national nature reserves, advise ministers and officials about various aspects of the natural environment and oversee the registration of sites of special scientific interest (SSSIs). With headquarters in England, Scotland and Wales and fifteen regional offices, they can deal with the country as a whole.

The majority of nature reserves in Britain are administered by local Naturalists' Trusts. The Society for the Promotion of Nature Conservation, The Green, Nettleham, Lincoln LN2 2NR, promotes the interests of nature conservation via local Naturalists' Trusts.

The Botanical Society of the British Isles, c/o Department of Botany, The British Museum of Natural History, Cromwell Road, London SW7 5BD, can help anyone interested in flowering plants, ferns and related groups, and other addresses to write to if you are interested in the countryside either in a general way or with something specific in mind are as follows:

Council For The Protection of Rural England, 4 Hobart Place, London SW1W 0HY.

National Trust, 42 Queen Anne's Gate, London SW1H 9AS.

National Trust for Scotland, 5 Charlotte Square, Edinburgh EH2 4DU.

Woodland Trust, Betterbrook, Harford, Ivybridge, Devon PL21 0JQ.

Friends of the Earth, 377 City Road, London EC1.

Wildlife, the Law and You warns that, unless you have a licence, you may not:

(*a*) intentionally pick, uproot or destroy any of the wild plants listed, or even collect their flowers and seeds;

(*b*) sell these plants or their seeds if taken from the wild;

(*c*) uproot *any* wild plant intentionally, except on your own land or with permission.

It is not illegal to pick most wild flowers or fruit (such as blackberries), but you should always leave enough to seed and for others to enjoy. You should not pick any wild flowers in a nature reserve.

The booklet lists the following specially protected wild plants:

Adder's-tongue spearwort
Alpine catchfly
Alpine gentian
Alpine sow-thistle
Alpine Woodsia
Bedstraw broomrape
Blue heath
Brown galingale
Cheddar pink
Childling pink
Diapensia
Dickie's bladder-fern
Downy woundwort
Drooping saxifrage
Early spider-orchid
Fen orchid
Fen violet
Field cow-wheat
Field eryngo
Field wormwood

Ghost orchid
Greater yellow-rattle
Jersey cudweed
Killarney fern
Lady's-slipper
Late spider-orchid
Least lettuce
Limestone woundwort
Lizard orchid
Military orchid
Monkey orchid
Norwegian sandwort
Oblong Woodsia
Oxtongue broomrape
Perennial knawel
Plymouth pear
Purple spurge
Red helleborine
Ribbon-leaved water-plantain
Rock cinquefoil

Rock sea-lavender (two rare species) Starved wood-sedge
Rough marsh-mallow Teesdale sandwort
Round-headed leek Thistle broomrape
Sea knotgrass Triangular club-rush
Sickle-leaved hare's-ear Tufted saxifrage
Small Alison Water germander
Small hare's-ear Whorled Solomon's-seal
Snowdon lily Wild cotoneaster
Spiked speedwell Wild gladiolus
Spring gentian Wood calamint
Starfruit

USA legislation

Legislation governing the picking, cutting or uprooting of wild plants or gathering their seeds, and the alteration and destruction of their habitat may vary from state to state throughout the USA. However, overall guidance can be obtained from the United States Fish and Wildlife Service, Washington DC 20240, USA.

Import and export of endangered plants is covered by specific legislation and must conform to regulations under the convention CITES, this being an acronym for the Convention on International Trade in Endangered Species (wild flora and fauna).

Certain plants have specific protection under state legislation and licences/permits to pick, gather or collect them for scientific research are issued for a limited time period only.

The movement, propagation, sale of or trade in certain plants is proscribed by federal law. Again, some states have minor differences and it is wise to acquaint yourself with state and federal rules before growing, harvesting or trading in plants that you know or suspect may be on this proscribed list, details of which can be obtained from the Fish and Wildlife Service.

A list of those plants determined by the Director of the Fish and Wildlife Service to be threatened in the USA is reproduced below. This information was kindly supplied by the United States Information Service, Embassy of the USA, 55–6 Upper Brook Street, London W1A 2LH, and is current at the date of publication of this book. No list is included of those plants proscribed by state or federal legislation.

USA: threatened plants

Species		Historic range
Scientific name	Common name	
Alismataceae – Water-plantain family: *Sagittaria fasciculata*	Bunched arrowhead	USA (NC, SC)
Asteraceae – Aster family: .		
Echinacea tennesseensis	Tennessee purple coneflower	USA (TN)
Lipochaeta venosa	None	USA (HI)
Berberidaceae – Barberry family: *Berberis sonnei*	Truckee barberry	USA (CA)
Betulaceae – Birch family: *Betula uber*	Virginia round-leaf birch	USA (VA)
Brassicaceae – Mustard family:		
Arabis mcdonaldiana	McDonald's rock-cress	USA (CA)
Erysimum capitatum var. *angustatum*	Contra Costa wallflower	do
Cactaceae – Cactus family:		
Ancistrocactus tobuschii (= *Echinocactus t., Mammillaria t.*)	Tobusch fishhook cactus	USA (TX)
Coryphantha minima (= *C. nellieae, Escobaria n., Mammillaria n.*)	Nellie cory cactus	do
Coryphantha ramillosa	Bunched cory cactus	USA (TX), Mexico (Coahuila)
Coryphantha sneedii var. *leei* (= *Escobaria l., Mammillaria l.*)	Lee pincushion cactus	USA (NM)
Coryphantha sneedii var. *sneedii* (= *Escobaria s., Mammillaria s.*)	Sneed pincushion cactus	USA (TX, NM)
Echinocactus horizonthalonius var. *nicholii*	Nichol's Turk's head cactus	USA (AZ)
Echinocereus engelmannii var. *purpureus*	Purple-spined hedgehog cactus	USA (UT)
Echinocereus kuenzleri (= *E. hempelii*)	Kuenzler hedgehog cactus	USA (NM)
Echinocereus lloydii (= *E. roetteri* var. *l.*)	Lloyd's hedgehog cactus	USA (TX)
Echinocereus reichenbachii var. *albertii* (= *E. melanocentrus*)	Black lace cactus	do
Echinocereus triglochidiatus var. *arizonicus* (= *E. arizonicus*)	Arizona hedgehog cactus	USA (AZ)
Echinocereus triglochidiatus var. *inermis* (= *E. coccineus*, var. *i., E. phoeniceus* var. *i.*)	Spineless hedgehog cactus	USA (CO, UT)
Echinocereus viridiflorus var. *davisii* (= *E. davisii*)	Davis' green pitaya	USA (TX)

Species		Historic range
Scientific name	Common name	
Neolloydia mariposensis (= *Echinocactus m.*, *Echinomastus m.*)	Lloyd's Mariposa cactus	do
Pediocactus bradyi (= *Toumeya b.*)	Brady pincushion cactus	USA (AZ)
Pediocactus knowltonii	Knowlton cactus	USA (NM, CO)
Pediocactus peeblesianus var. *peeblesianus* (= *Echinocactus p., Navajoa p., Toumeya p., Utahia p.*)	Peebles Navajo cactus	USA (AZ)
Pediocactus sileri (= *Echinocactus s., Utahia s.*)	Siler pincushion cactus	USA (AZ, UT)
Sclerocactus glaucus (= *Echinocactus g., E. subglaucus, E. whipplei* var. *g., Pediocactus g., S. franklinii*)	Uinta Basin hookless cactus	USA (CO, UT)
Sclerocactus mesae-verdae (= *Coloradoa m., Echinocactus m., Pediocactus m.*)	Mesa Verde cactus	USA (CO, NM)
Sclerocactus wrightiae (= *Pediocactus w.*)	Wright fishhook cactus	USA (UT)
Cistaceae – Rockrose family: *Hudsonia montana*	Mountain golden heather	USA (NC)
Crassulaceae – Stonecrop family: *Dudleya traskiae*	Santa Barbara Island liveforever	USA (CA)
Cupressaceae – Cypress family: *Fitzroya cupressoides*	Chilean false larch (= alerce)	Chile, Argentina
Ericaceae – Heath family:		
Arctostaphylos hookeri ssp. *ravenii*	Raven's manzanita	USA (CA)
Rhododendron chapmanii	Chapman rhododendron	USA (FL)
Euphorbiaceae – Spurge family: *Euphorbia skottsbergii* var. *kalaeloana*	'Ewa Plains 'akoko	USA (HI)
Fabaceae – Pea family:		
Astragalus perianus	Rydberg milk-vetch	USA (UT)
Baptisia arachnifera	Hairy rattleweed	USA (GA)
Lotus dendroideus (= *scoparius*) ssp. *traskiae*	San Clemente Island broom	USA (CA)
Vicia menziesii	Hawaiian vetch	USA (HI)
Hydrophyllaceae – Waterleaf family:		
Phacelia argillacea	None	USA (UT)
Phacelia formosula	North Park phacelia	USA (CO)
Lamiaceae – Mint family:		
Haplostachys haplostachya var. *angustifolia*	None	USA (HI)

Species		Historic range
Scientific name	Common name	
Hedeoma apiculatum	Mint family – McKittrick pennyroyal	USA (TX, NM)
Hedeoma todsenii	Todsenis pennyroyal	USA (NM)
Pogogyne abramsii	San Diego mesa mint	USA (CA)
Stenogyne angustifolia var. *angustifolia*	None	USA (HI)
Liliaceae – Lily family:		
Harperocallis flava	Harper's beauty	USA (FL)
Trillium persistens	Persistent trillium	USA (GA, SC)
Malvaceae – Mallow family:		
Callirhoe scabriuscula	Texas poppy-mallow	USA (TX)
Kokia cookei	Cooke's kokio	USA (HI)
Malacothamnus clementinus	San Clemente Island bush-mallow	USA (CA)
Nyctaginaceae – Four-o'clock family: *Mirabilis macfarlanei*	MacFarlane's four-o'clock	USA (ID, OR)
Onagraceae – Evening-primrose family:		
Oenothera avita ssp. *eurekensis*	Eureka Valley evening-primrose	USA (CA)
Oenothera deltoides ssp. *howellii*	Antioch Dunes evening-primrose	do
Orchidaceae – Orchid family:		
Spiranthese parksii	Navasota ladies'-tresses	USA (Texas)
Isotria medeoloides	Small whorled pogonia	Canada (Ontario) and USA (CT, IL, MA, MD, ME, MI, MO, NC, NH, NJ, NY, PA, RI, SC, VA, VT)
Papaveraceae – Poppy family: *Arctomecon humilis*	Dwarf bear-poppy	USA (UT)
Pinaceae – Pine family: *Abies guatemalensis*	Guatemalan fir (= pinabete)	Mexico, Guatemala, Honduras, El Salvador
Poaceae – Grass family:		
Orcuttia mucronata	Solano (= Crampton's Orcutt) grass	USA (CA)
Swallenia alexandrae	Eureka Dune grass	do
Zizania texana	Texas wild-rice	USA (TX)
Polygonaceae – Buckwheat family: *Eriogonum gypsophilum*	Gypsum wild buckwheat	USA (NM)

Species		Historic
Scientific name	Common name	range
Ranunculaceae – Buttercup family:		
Aconitum noveboracense	Northern wild monkshood	USA (IA, NY, OH, WI)
Delphinium kinkiense	San Clemente Island larkspur	USA (CA)
Rosaceae – Rose family: *Potentilla robbinsiana*	Robbins cinquefoil	USA (NH, VT)
Sarraceniaceae – Pitcher plant family: *Sarracenia oreophila*	Green pitcher plant	USA (AL, GA)
Scrophulariaceae – Snapdragon family:		
Castilleja grisea	San Clemente Island Indian paintbrush	USA (CA)
Cordylanthus maritimus ssp. *maritimus*	Salt marsh bird's beak	USA (CA), Mexico (Baja California)
Pedicularis furbishiae	Furbish lousewort	USA (ME), Canada (New Brunswick)

Bibliography

BRYAN, Felicity, *The Town Gardener's Companion*. Penguin Books Ltd, 1983.

CONWAY, David, *The Magic of Herbs*. Readers Union Group of Bookclubs, Newton Abbot 1975.

DREWITT, F. Dawtrey, *The Romance of The Apothecaries' Garden at Chelsea*. Chapman & Dodd Ltd, 1922.

EAGLE, Robert, *Herbs, Useful Plants*. BBC, 1981

FLUCK, Prof. Hans, *Medicinal Plants*, trans. Prof. J. M. Rowson. W. Foulsham & Co. Ltd, Slough, 1976.

FRITSCH, F. E. and SALISBURY, E. J., *An Introduction to the Study of Plants*. G. Bell & Sons Ltd, 1935.

GLOB, P. V., *The Bog People*. Faber Paperbacks, 1977.

GORDON, Lesley, *Green Magic*. Ebury Press, Exeter, 1977.

GRIGSON, Geoffrey, *A Dictionary of English Plant Names*. Allen Lane, 1974.

— *A Herbal of All Sorts*. Phoenix House, 1959.

HARRIS, Ben Charles, *Eat The Weeds*. Keats Publishing Inc., New Canaan, Connecticut, 1973.

HARVEY, Jack, *Herbs*. Macdonald Educational, 1976.

HOLE, Christina, *English Custom and Usage*. B. T. Batsford Ltd, 1941.

HUXLEY, Anthony, *The Penguin Encyclopedia of Gardening*. Penguin Books Ltd, 1981.

JEKYLL, G. and JONES, S. R., *Old English Household Life*. B. T. Batsford Ltd, 2nd printing 1944.

JOHNS, Rev. C. A., *Flowers of the Field*. General Literature Committee, London, 1910.

KADANS, Joseph M., *Encyclopedia of Medicinal Herbs*. Thorsons Publishers Ltd, Wellingborough, 1983.

KEBLE MARTIN, W., *The Concise British Flora in Colour*. Sphere Books, 1978.

LE STRANGE, Richard, *A History of Herbal Plants*. Angus & Robertson Publishers, 1977.

LEVY, J. de Bairacli, *Herbal Handbook for Everyone*. Faber & Faber Ltd, 1966.

LOEWENFELD, Claire and BACK, Philippa, *The Complete Book of Herbs & Spices*. David & Charles, 1974.

LOEWENFELD, Claire and BACK, Phillipa, with BOSANQUET, Patience, *Britain's Wild Larder*. David & Charles, 1980.

LUCAS, Richard, *Secrets of the Chinese Herbalists*. Thorsons Publishers Ltd, 1977.

MABEY, Richard, *The Common Ground*. Hutchinson, 1980.

MCCLINTOCK, David and FITTER, R. S. R., *Collins Pocket Guide to Wild Flowers*. Collins, 11th printing 1978.

MASSINGHAM, Betty, *A Century of Gardeners*. Faber & Faber, 1982.

MESSEGUÉ, Maurice with PETER, Madeleine, *A Kitchen Herbal (Making the most of herbs for cookery and health)*. Collins, 1983.

MITCHELL, Alan and WILKINSON, John, *The Trees of Britain and Northern Europe*. Collins, 1982.

NATURE CONSERVANCY COUNCIL (Report Booklets), London 1982–3.

NILSSON, Sven and PERSSON, Olle, illustrated by Bo Mossberg, *Fungi of Northern Europe (Parts 1 and 2)*. Penguin Nature Guides, 1978.

OWEN, Gale R., *Rites and Religions of the Anglo-Saxons*. David & Charles, 1981.

PALAISEUL, Jean, *Grandmother's Secrets*. Penguin, 1973.

Pharmaceutical Press, *The Pharmaceutical Pocket Book*, London, 1960.

PHILLIPS, Roger, *Trees in Britain, Europe and North America*. Pan Books, 1978.

— *Wild Flowers of Britain*. Pan Books, 1977.

POLUNIN, Oleg, *The Concise Flowers of Europe*. Oxford University Press, 1972.

POTTERTON, David, ed., *Culpeper's Colour Herbal*. W. Foulsham & Co. Ltd, 1983.

ROSE, Francis, *The Observer's Book of Grasses, Sedges and Rushes*. Frederick Warne & Co. Ltd, 1974.

SANDERS, T. W., *The Alphabet of Gardening*. W. H. & L. Collingridge, 1927.

SANECKI, Kay, *The Complete Book of Herbs*. Macdonald, 1974.

SKENE, MacGregor, *A Flower Book for the Pocket*. Oxford University Press, 1941.

THOMPSON, C. J. S., *The Mystic Mandrake*. Rider & Co., 1934.

THOMPSON, William A. R., MD, *Herbs that Heal*. Adam & Charles Black, 1976.

TRITTON, S. M., *Amateur Wine-Making*. Faber & Faber, 1968.

URQUHART, Judy, *Living Off Nature*. Penguin Books, 1982.

Botanical Names

Acacia senegal, Acacia vera acacia
Achillea millefolium yarrow
Aesculus hippocastanum horse chestnut
Agrimonia eupatoria agrimony
Ajuga reptans bugle
Allium porrum leek
Allium sativum garlic
Alnus glutinosa alder
Althaea officinalis mallow, marsh
Althaea rosea hollyhock
Anemone hepatica, Anemone nemorosa, Anemone pulsatilla anemone
Angelica archangelica, Angelica officinalis angelica
Anthyllis vulneraria kidney vetch
Aquilegia vulgaris aquilegia
Arctium lappa burdock
Aristolochia clematitis birthwort
Armoracia rusticana horseradish
Arnica montana arnica
Artemisia absinthium absinthe
Artemisia dracunculus tarragon
Artemisia vulgare mugwort
Arum maculatum wild arum
Asparagus officinalis asparagus
Atropa belladonna belladonna/ deadly nightshade

Ballota nigra black horehound
Bellis perennis daisy
Betula pendula silver birch
Bidens connata (swamp beggar's tick) see under water agrimony
Bidens tripartita water agrimony
Borago officinalis borage
Brassica oleracea cabbage
Bryonia dioica white bryony

Calendula officinalis marigold
Capsella bursa-pastoris shepherd's purse
Carlina vulgaris carline thistle
Carum carvi caraway
Centaurea jacea (knapwort) see under knapweed
Centaurea nigra knapweed
Centaurea scabiosa (large knapweed) see under knapweed
Centaurium erythraea centaury
Chenopodium bonus henricus good king henry
Chrysanthemum parthenium feverfew
Chrysanthemum segetum (corn marigold) see under marigold
Clematis vitalba old man's beard
Convallaria majalis lily of the valley

Cydonia oblonga   quince
Cytisus scoparius   broom

Daucus carota   carrot

Equisetum arvense   horsetail
Erigeron acre   fleabane

Ficus carica   fig
Filipendula ulmaria
   meadowsweet
Fragaria vesca   wild strawberry
Frangula alnus   alder buckthorn
Fraxinus excelsior   ash, common
Fumaria officinalis   fumitory

Galium aparine   cleavers/
   goosegrass
Galium odoratum   sweet
   woodruff
Geum urbanum   herb bennet
Glechoma hederacea   ground ivy
Glycyrrhiza glabra   liquorice

Hedera helix   ivy, common
Helianthus annuus   sunflower
Hieracium pilosella   mouse-ear
   hawkweed
Humulus lupulus   hops
Hypericum perforatum   St John's
   wort
Hyssopus officinalis   hyssop

Inula helenium   elecampane
Iris foetidissima, Iris pseudacorus
   iris

Juglans regia   walnut
Juniperus communis   juniper

Lactuca sativa   lettuce
Lactuca virosa (prickly lettuce)
   see under lettuce
Linum usitatissimum   flax
Lonicera periclymenum
   honeysuckle

Malus pumila (apple)   see under
   crab apple
Malus sylvestris   crab apple
Malva moschata (musk mallow),
   Malva sylvestris (common
   mallow)   see under mallow,
   marsh
*Matricaria chamomilla, Matricaria
   recutita*   chamomile
Matricaria maritima (scentless
   mayweed)   see under
   chamomile
Medicago sativa   alfalfa/sweet
   lucerne
Melilotus officinalis   melilot
Melissa officinalis   lemon balm
Mentha × piperata   peppermint
Mentha spicata   spearmint
Myrrhis odorata   sweet cecily

Nepeta cataria × faassenii
   catmint
Nuphar lutea (yellow lily)   see
   under water lily
Nymphaea alba   water lily

Ocimum basilicum   basil
Oenothera biennis   evening
   primrose
Ophioglossum vulgatum   adder's
   tongue
*Origanum marjorana, Origanum
   vulgare*   marjoram

*Panax quinquefolius, Panax
   schinseng*   ginseng
Papaver rhoeas   poppy
Papaver somniferum (opium
   poppy)   see under poppy
Pimpinella anisum   aniseed
Plantago major   plantain
Polygonum aviculare   knotgrass
Potentilla anserina   silverweed
Potentilla erecta (tormentil),
   Potentilla reptans (cinquefoil)
   see under silverweed
Primula officinalis, Primula veris
   cowslip

Primula vulgaris (primrose)   see
  under cowslip
Pulicaria dysenterica   fleabane

*Rheum officinale, Rheum
  palmatum*   rhubarb
Rhus radicans (poison ivy)   see
  under ground ivy
Rosa canina   dog rose
Rubus fruticosus   blackberry
Rubus idaeus   raspberry
Ruta graveolens   rue, common

*Salix alba, Salix caprea, Salix
  fragilis, Salix species*   willow
Salvia officinalis   sage
Sambucus ebulus   dane wort/
  dwarf elder
Sambucus nigra   elder
Sanguisorba minor (salad burnet)
  see under great burnet
Sanguisorba officinalis   great
  burnet
Saponaria officinalis   soapwort
Senecio vulgaris   groundsel
Silybum marianum   milk thistle
Solanum dulcamara   woody
  nightshade

Solanum tuberosum   potato
Sphagnum cymbifolium
  sphagnum moss
Stachys officinalis   betony
Stachys palustris   marsh
  woundwort
Symphytum officinale   comfrey

Tamus communis   black bryony
Taraxacum officinale   dandelion
*Thymus serpyllum, Thymus
  vulgaris*   thyme
Tilia europaea   lime/linden tree
Tropaeolum majus   nasturtium
Tussilago farfara   coltsfoot

Ulmus campestris   elm
Urtica dioica   nettle

Valeriana officinalis   valerian
Verbascum thapsus   Aaron's rod
Verbena officinalis   vervain
Viola canina (dog violet)   see
  under violet, sweet
Viola odorata   violet, sweet
Viola tricolor   heartsease
Viscum album   mistletoe

Zingiber offinale   ginger

Index of Uses

Only those uses of practical modern-day value are listed. Please read the safety warnings given in the Author's Note and under the individual entries.

Abcess   flax, ivy
Anaemia   blackberry, carrot
Arthritis   ash, meadowsweet, wild strawberry
Asthma   hyssop

Bites   broom
Bladder infection   horsetail
Blister   cabbage, old man's beard
Boils   arnica, carrot, elm, flax, horseradish, ivy, mallow (marsh), mallow (musk), potato, violet (sweet), water lily
Broken bones   comfrey
Bronchitis   elecampane, ground ivy, honeysuckle, horsetail, hyssop, lettuce, liquorice, tormentil (see silverweed), wild strawberry
Bruises   alder, arnica, bugle, comfrey, cowslip, daisy, kidney vetch, nettle, primrose (see cowslip), violet (dog)
Burns (scalds/sunburn)   carrot, great burnet, leek, mallow

(marsh), nettle, St John's wort, water lily

Catarrh   basil, horseradish, knapweed
Chilblains   adder's tongue, figs
Colds   basil, bugle, catmint, coltsfoot, elder, feverfew, honeysuckle, horseradish, hyssop, lime/linden tree, marjoram, nettle, raspberry, thyme, willow
Coughs   Aaron's rod, acacia, apple (see crab apple), black horehound, cabbage, catmint, coltsfoot, cowslip, elder, fig, garlic, honeysuckle, horseradish, horsetail, hyssop, leek, lime/linden tree, liquorice, mallow (musk), marjoram, nasturtium, nettle, primrose (see cowslip), sunflower, thyme, violet (sweet)
Cuts   adder's tongue, agrimony, bugle, cleavers, coltsfoot, comfrey, flax, great burnet, ground ivy, herb bennet, kidney vetch, knotgrass, marigold, marsh woundwort, peppermint, plantain, potato, St John's wort, shepherd's

purse, sphagnum moss, thyme, violet (sweet)

Cystitis   agrimony, knotgrass, mallow (marsh), silverweed, tormentil (see silverweed), wild strawberry

Diarrhoea   apple (see crab apple), elm, fleabane, knotgrass, leek, lettuce, lime/linden tree, silverweed, tormentil (see silverweed)

Digestion, aid to, and digestive ailments   absinthe, acacia, agrimony, alfalfa, angelica, aniseed, basil, blackberry, caraway, carline thistle, centaury, cowslip, dandelion, elm, flax, fleabane, ginger, herb bennet, hollyhock, horseradish, knapweed, knotgrass, lemon balm, mallow (marsh), marigold, melilot, peppermint, poppy, primrose (see cowslip), quince, raspberry, rhubarb, rue, sage, St John's wort, spearmint, thyme, tormentil (see silverweed), vervain, walnut

Dyes and pigments   acacia, agrimony, betony, elder, knapweed, knotgrass, marigold

External parasites   fleabane, leek, rue, sweet cecily, sweet woodruff

Gastric upsets   agrimony, elecampane, mallow (common), nasturtium, peppermint, St John's wort, walnut, wild strawberry

Gout   ash, comfrey, dandelion, hyssop, juniper, meadowsweet, nettle, silver birch, wild strawberry

Grazes   agrimony, bugle, cleavers, coltsfoot, comfrey, great burnet, ground ivy, herb bennet, marigold, marsh woundwort, peppermint, plantain, potato, St John's wort, shepherd's purse, thyme, violet (dog), water lily

Haemorrhoids   horse chestnut, silverweed, yarrow

Hair care   chamomile, nasturtium, quince, thyme

Hangover   ginger

Hay fever   tormentil (see silverweed)

Headache (migraine)   Aaron's rod, angelica, basil, betony, feverfew, meadowsweet, vervain, willow

Insect repellant   absinthe, elder, walnut

Internal parasites   absinthe, broom, garlic, walnut

Intestinal ailments/bowel disorders   honeysuckle, quince, rhubarb, sage

Jaundice   broom, spearmint, vervain

Kidney ailments   carrot, chamomile, dandelion, horsetail, silver birch, vervain

Laxative   acacia, ash, elder, fig, flax, liquorice, quince, rhubarb, violet (sweet)

Liver disorders   chamomile

Menstrual disorders (and pain)   chamomile, elecampane, ginger, groundsel, lemon balm, marigold, melilot, pasque flower (see anemone), St John's wort, shepherd's purse, sweet woodruff, tormentil (see silverweed), water agrimony, yarrow

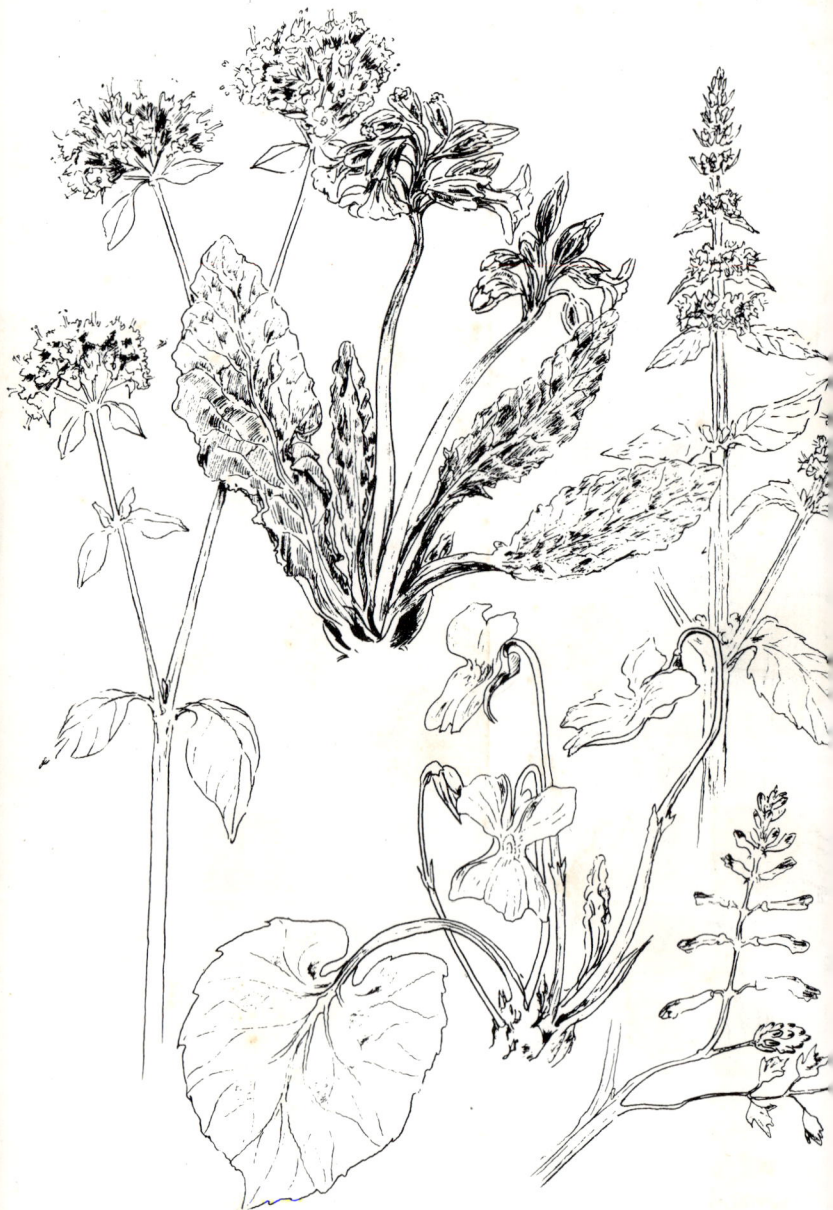